PENGUIN BOOKS

RATING THE EXERCISES

Charles T. Kuntzleman has served as the national director of the Y.M.C.A. Fitness Finders Program, conducting hundreds of workshops across the United States and in Canada. The author of many books and articles on fitness, diet, and health, he lives in Michigan with his wife and five children.

The editors of *Consumer Guide®*, which is published in Chicago, are well known for their many excellent self-help books, including *Rating the Diets* and *The Whole House Catalog*.

RATING THE EXERCISES

by Charles T. Kuntzleman
and THE EDITORS
of CONSUMER GUIDE®

PENGUIN BOOKS

Penguin Books Ltd, Harmondsworth,
Middlesex, England
Penguin Books, 625 Madison Avenue,
New York, New York 10022, U.S.A.
Penguin Books Australia Ltd, Ringwood,
Victoria, Australia
Penguin Books Canada Limited, 2801 John Street,
Markham, Ontario, Canada L3R 1B4
Penguin Books (N.Z.) Ltd, 182–190 Wairau Road,
Auckland 10, New Zealand

First published in the United States of America by
William Morrow and Company, Inc., 1978
Published in Penguin Books 1980

Copyright © Publications International Limited, 1978
All rights reserved

LIBRARY OF CONGRESS CATALOGING IN PUBLICATION DATA
Kuntzleman, Charles T.
Rating the exercises
Includes bibliographical references and index.
1. Exercise. 2. Physical fitness. I. Consumer guide. II. Title.
RA781.K85   1980   613.7'1   79-21477
ISBN 0 14 00.5191 0

Printed in the United States of America by
Offset Paperback Mfrs., Inc., Dallas, Pennsylvania
Set in Times Roman

CONTENTS

CONTENTS

INTRODUCTION

WE AMERICANS ARE THE MOST PAMPERED PEOPLE ON EARTH. Almost every family has two cars—some have three. We have at our disposal hundreds of laborsaving devices to make our work easier and perhaps more enjoyable. Modern conveniences have eliminated hard physical labor from our lives. Some farmers, nurses, and construction workers may protest that statement, but let's face it. Many of the most active occupations and life-styles of today would have been considered just mildly active one hundred years ago.

Modern technology may have made our life easier, but it has also made us less healthy. Almost one million Americans die of heart disease each year. One tenth of all Americans suffer from hypertension. And over one-half of the adult population carries too much weight or struggles to keep it under control.

We worry about our sedentary life-style and realize that our way of life may be jeopardizing our health. But what really bothers us is that we don't *look* good. As we grow older we start to lose our attractive, lean look. Our hips spread, our waistlines expand, and our arms look flabby. We get upset because we want to look fit, trim, and healthy. That way we will have a better self-image, be admired, and get to the top more quickly.

Oh, how we want to be fit. The problem is that few of us want to take the time to be trim and healthy. We look for an easy way. Perhaps if we cinch in our waist and hips with girdles, hide our bay windows with Brooks Brothers suits, and "face-lift" sagging facial muscles we will look better. Those of us who are more actively inclined jump from one fitness bandwagon to another—isometrics, aerobics, Total Fitness, etc. The "experts"—some legitimate and some phony—tell us they can solve our fitness problems.

Browse in any bookstore and you'll see that plenty of advice is available on exercise to strengthen your heart, stretch your body, build your biceps, and control your fat. Some plans promise instant fitness; others emphasize a painless approach. Some tell you to increase your pulse rate; others tell you not to waste a heartbeat. The experts make their pitch on TV talk shows and through the news media, telling you theirs is the only way. They have found the secret to real total fitness.

Obviously, they can't all be right. They contradict each other, leaving you frustrated. You may even be angry because what the experts are saying doesn't match your own experience.

Who is going to lead you out of this maze of fitness confusion? Who is going to help you decide which program to follow to effectively control body weight, firm up muscles, strengthen hearts, and stretch bodies?

Until now there has been no objective guide to help you decide which program is best. Every expert has a book, and each book has its critics. Until now there has been no tool to help you analyze the programs and the fitness needs of your body.

Rating the Exercises does all this, and more. Here in one book is everything you need to look critically at each program now on the market and the new ones to come. These tools are adaptable; they will last and last, though new experts and programs come and go.

In *Rating the Exercises, Consumer Guide®* presents the hard facts about fitness. After reading these pages, the facts should stand out boldly and clearly, and you should be able to make the appropriate decisions in pursuit of fitness.

This book rates the current crop of fitness programs and helps you determine how much exercise you need. Consideration is also given to many oft-asked questions: What are the real benefits of exercise? What are the advantages of yoga, isometrics, running, and favorite sports? What are the disadvantages? Can certain exercises hurt rather than help? Is there such a thing as a "perfect exercise" or sport? How much exercise is enough? Must a person exercise every day? Can exercise improve our cardiac health, sex life, and body contours?

After analyzing all the research, talking to the experts, and evaluating the pros and cons of exercise, *Consumer Guide®* concludes that there is a "best exercise," a type that will be good for your health and for your looks. The "best" is cardiovascular exercise, the kind that gets your heart and lungs working harder. It can be any of many different activities that are characterized by repeatedly and vigorously moving the major muscles of your body for an extended period of time.

The ratings assigned in this book are based on our conclusion that cardiovascular type exercise is best for heart, muscles, body weight, and appearance. In other words, to be rated highly in this book, an exercise program must have a proper cardiovascular element. Programs that emphasize flexibility or strength cannot, therefore, receive the highest rating, no matter how effective the program is in pursuing its own primary goal. The most important muscle of one's body is the heart, and a good fitness program must recongize this fact. Cardiovascular exercise cannot be neglected.

Rating the Exercises describes and rates current exercise programs, but it does not replace the books or organized groups that supply you with the tools for following them.

These books and organizations offer guidelines and inspiration to help you start on a program.

Once you have started, keep *Rating the Exercises* handy as a reference. The information it contains will not lose validity. As your fitness level improves, you may want to change your program. Simply pick up *Rating the Exercises* and thumb through it for the information you need to move on. This should be a well-used book. Use it to start the process that will help you reach the fitness level you want and then help you stay there.

RATING
THE
EXERCISES

1

THE ACTIVITY EXPLOSION

No doubt about it. America is fitness conscious.

Listen to the talk at coffee breaks, parties, anywhere people get together to chat. We're worried about sagging body contours, poor muscle tone, listlessness, lack of energy, being "out of shape." We boast of miles jogged, analyze tennis techniques, lament our latest golf score, report on our bowling record.

The concern for physical fitness is reflected in the unprecedented boom in the sporting goods industry. Sales have jumped dramatically during the past few years. Americans spent over $418 million for tennis equipment in 1974, $555 million in 1975, and $666 million in 1976. Ski equipment also showed a tremendous upsurge. In 1974, more than $343 million was spent; in 1975, $379 million; and in 1976, $421 million.[1] Moreover, as of January 1, 1975, 3.5 million swimming pools were constructed in and above the ground. That's one pool for every twenty U.S. families![2]

The health-club industry is also experiencing a boom. It has been estimated that about three million Americans are paying more than $300 a year to belong to a commercial health club.[3] Glenn Swengros, Vice President of European Health Spas—the nation's largest chain of commercial gymnasiums—reports that their spas attract more than 12,000 new

13

members a month. The National YMCA reports that over the past several years the Y conducted almost 300,000 different physical education activities for eight million registered participants.[4] Interestingly, about two million of these participants were women.

Exercise equipment is bullish. Every day thousands of dollars are spent on treadmills, mini gymnasiums, stationary bicycles, weights, exercise wheels, and waist trimmers—a range of items tailored to fit almost every type of pocketbook.

Another sign of the intense interest in fitness is the increasing output of the publishing industry on the subject. We Americans gobble up exercise books at a rate that brings joy to their publishers' hearts. Scan any popular newsstand and you'll find a mind-boggling array of materials on exercise as a means of achieving good health and overall well-being, weight control—and, yes, better sex.

From the top level of the U.S. government itself came the 1973 report by the President's Council on Physical Fitness and Sports saying that 55 percent—that's 60 million—of our adult population engages in one or more forms of exercise. Almost 44 million walk, 22 million bowl, 18 million bicycle, 14 million do calisthenics, 10 million golf, and 6.5 million jog.[5]

EXPLOSION OR ILLUSION?

But despite all the attention focused on fitness, the number of Americans who exercise on a *regular* basis is low.

The President's Council has defined "regular exercise" as participation in an activity at least three times a week. By this standard, the Council's report shows that a large percentage of our adult population does *not* exercise sufficiently. Most people participate only two days a week or less. In fact, 90 percent of the bowlers, tennis players, and others who engage in participatory sports; 83 percent of the golfers; 70 percent of the swimmers; 60 percent of the bicyclists; 50 percent of the joggers; 33 percent of the weight lifters; 30 percent of the walkers; and 23 percent of the people who do calisthenics "do their thing" less frequently than three times a week.[6]

FIGURE 1 / EXERCISE IN THE UNITED STATES

ACTIVITY	PERCENTAGE PARTICIPATING	NUMBERS PARTICIPATING
Walking	40%	43.6 million
Bowling	20	21.8
Bicyling	17	18.5
Swimming	13	14.2
Calisthenics	13	14.2
Golf	9	9.8
Softball	8.5	9.3
Jogging	6	6.5
Tennis	6	6.5
Volleyball	5	5.4
Water Skiing	5	5.4
Weight Training	3	3.3
Skiing	2	2.2

Based on "National Adult Physical Fitness Survey," *The President's Council on Physical Fitness and Sports Newsletter*, May 1973.

Thus, when the President's Council applies its three-times-a-week standard, it turns out that only thirty million adult Americans exercise regularly, which is only about 28 percent of our population.[7] Furthermore, 45 percent of the population gets no exercise at all!

Other experts [8] see the situation as being even more dismal. Some believe that recent statistics on the Canadian population are probably closer to the truth about Americans. According to a 1975 study, only 20 percent of the Canadian population engages in some form of physical activity such as walking for pleasure, jogging, hiking, or other exercise.[9]

Dr. Kenneth Cooper, M.D., of *Aerobics* fame, is convinced that the President's Council's estimate that thirty million Americans exercise regularly is an enormous exaggeration. "It's probably more like ten to fifteen million—probably less," he says. "And even these people aren't all exercising regularly." [10]

Exercise physiologist Dr. Paul Lessick, Ph.D., is even more pessimistic. He doesn't accept the President's Council's estimate that 55 percent of Americans engage in at least some exercise. Furthermore, applying his own more demanding standards, Dr. Lessick concluded that only 5 to 7 percent of the population surveyed by the Council was getting the proper kind and amount of exercise. Dr. Elsworth R. Buskirk, Ph.D.,[11] director of the Noll Laboratory for Human Performance Research at the Pennsylvania State University, concurs. He estimates that less than 5 percent of the general population now exercises regularly.

The most skeptical of all, however, is Dr. Joseph Ahrends, M.D., a cardiologist specializing in preventive medicine. He has stated that "past the age of thirty-five less than two percent of American males and less than one percent of American females are physically fit." [12] In other words, only 1 to 2 percent of the adult population past the age of thirty-five are getting adequate exercise.

But we're not happy about our inactivity; we do care. We know we *ought* to be exercising. We know we feel better and function more efficiently when we're "in good shape." We plan to be active, buy the equipment, read (or at least purchase) the books and magazines that promise to help us carry out a physical exercise program. But what happens to our good intentions?

AMERICA'S MECHANIZED SOCIETY

The accelerated interest in and worry over exercise is a response to the changing face of everyday American life. The modern industrial age has produced countless benefits in consumer goods, production, transportation, communications, medicine, etc. It has also resulted in life and work patterns that are virtually sedentary.

Centuries ago, most people lived by strength and endurance. Every day brought tasks that required vigorous and dynamic physical action. Success and even survival meant being able to run fast and long and to strike hard if attacked. Physical fitness was necessary. Just three or four generations ago, most of the U.S. population lived in small towns or on farms and had to do a good bit of walking. Even city dwellers walked a great deal—footing it to work, to the market, to friends, to parties and celebrations. Walking to and from an evening's entertainment was considered part of the entertainment.

Two-story houses were the rule, so there was a lot of running up and down stairs. Yards were cared for with scythes and hand mowers. Snow was shoveled; leaves were raked. Wood had to be cut with an ax and stacked for the fireplace. Clothes were scrubbed clean on a washboard, hung out to dry, and then pressed with an iron that weighed seven pounds or more.

About fifty years ago, a dramatic change began to take place. The "machine age" arrived and rapidly changed America's working habits. As work became more and more mechanized, people were left with less and less physical work to do. Consequently, the average adult American today hardly has to move a muscle.

Most of us live in one of our country's urban or suburban areas. Instead of walking to a store two or four blocks away, we drive there in a car. We use an elevator or escalator to get from one floor of a building to another. Grass is cut with a sit-and-ride mower, leaves and snow are sucked up by power-driven vacuum devices, and we need only flick a switch to heat our homes.

Even our recreation has become mechanized. Speedboats,

snowmobiles, and golf in a golf cart are typical forms of recreation. Our leisure time on Saturday or Sunday is spent watching football and sporting events on TV.

At work we operate machines of all kinds—typewriters, factory machines, trucks. We press buttons, turn knobs, flip switches, punch keys, turn wheels, and pull levers. We are nearly always sitting—at desks and tables, behind the wheel, at our machine. We supervise, manage, steer, talk, advise, refill, regulate, but few of us ever lift, push, stretch, or strain.

One well-known expert in sports medicine, Dr. Donald Cooper, M.D., athletic team physician at Oklahoma State University, estimates that "only two percent of American adults get enough exercise in their workaday world, when one hundred years ago at least fifty percent got sufficient exercise from the job."

It's up to us, then, to deliberately introduce physical activity into our daily routine. Exercise is no longer naturally integrated into a normal day; we have to put it there.

This is difficult. The decision has to be conscious, the time has to be found, and, if you desire, the facilities sought out or equipment obtained. You have to do these things in addition to your daily work and personal routine. In fact, you probably have to make room for them by eliminating some other leisure-time activity. It's no wonder so many people fall short.

THE RISKS OF INACTIVITY

Our instinctive enjoyment of exercise is a clue to its biological importance. The evidence of science and statistics tells us that exercise is not just a pleasure. It is essential.

The "good life" our forebears diligently strove to achieve has given us many benefits, but fitness is not one of them. Recent statistics reveal that we are among the fattest and sickest peoples on this earth. Our sedentary life-style has contributed to a host of ailments that affect our health, vitality, vigor, and productivity.

We're tired before the middle of the day, our waistline expands, our weight escalates, we suffer heart attacks while shoveling snow, we're short of breath after two flights of stairs, we're uptight, we're nervous, and we suffer from mysterious aches and pains.

Doctors Hans Kraus, M.D., and Wilhelm Raab, M.D.,[13] have coined the term "hypokinetic [caused by insufficient motion] diseases" to describe the spectrum of illnesses and disorders that may be caused or influenced by our sedentary life-style. They believe this life-style interferes with the biological function of action and that this interference is physically damaging to humans.

The concept of hypokinetic disease is based on a view of the human body as being essentially active and dynamic in nature. Kraus and Raab, however, contend that the natural physical response gets bottled up, and that this very bottling up causes tension which, if not relieved, can lead to emotional or physical illness. Diseases resulting from (or aggravated by) stress include various metabolic ailments (obesity is most common), endocrine malfunctions, gastrointestinal upsets and malfunctions, degenerative cardiovascular diseases, and musculoskeletal dysfunction. Emotional disorders include neurosis, anxiety, depression, and various compulsions. Each of these ailments—physical and emotional—can cause more tension. And so the cycle whirls and widens.

In 1971, Dr. Jesse Steinfeld, M.D., then Surgeon General of the U.S. Public Health Service, lamented the lack of exercise in everyday modern life:

> Instead of man spending most of his time trying to get his food—in order to live—by chasing after animals, climbing trees, running away from other animals that might want to eat him, . . . we have automobiles and elevators, trains and planes, motorcycles, bicycles and all sorts of things. . . . Accordingly, we must

exercise if we are to preserve our health—we will sleep better, eat better, digest our food better.... People who are in good physical condition even enjoy sex more. If that isn't a motivating factor, I don't know what is.[14]

Failure to use the body's strength and endurance is, then, contrary to our basic need to move. Our muscles, which constitute a major portion of our body weight, serve many more functions than locomotion. In addition to having direct and indirect influence on our circulatory, metabolic, and endocrine systems, and on our bones, posture, and body position, our muscles serve as an outlet for emotions and a means for nervous responses. We must use them to preserve a healthy balance between our mental and physical capacities.

EXERCISE AND HEALTH: THE EVIDENCE

A growing body of contemporary research has been pointing to the value of exercise in preventing, retarding, or modifying various diseases and disorders. The range of disorders thought to be related to underactivity is broad and perhaps startling. Later chapters will take up the most important developments in detail; here we mention each briefly to show how far-reaching and all-pervasive are the benefits of regular exercise.

Coronary Artery Disease. The American Heart Association lists eleven factors that predispose a person to heart disease—and lack of exercise is one of them.[15] Endurance exercise may also play a role in reducing several of the other risk factors, including stress, high blood pressure, and elevated blood fats. At this date, according to Doctors Samuel Fox, M.D., and William Haskell, Ph.D., there is not enough evidence to prove that exercise *prevents* heart disease, but it certainly is considered by many to be a promising field for investigation and a prudent practice for most people to follow.[16]

Overweight and Obesity. Exercise is an important part of many weight-reducing programs. The link between inactivity and excess fat is widely recognized. Experts agree with Dr. Jean Mayer, world-famous nutritionist:

> I am convinced that inactivity is the most important factor explaining the frequency of "creeping" overweight in modern societies. Our bodies' regulation of food intake was just not designed for the highly mechanized condition of modern life. . . . Adapting to these conditions without developing obesity means either that the individual will have to step up his activity or that he will be mildly or acutely hungry all his life.[17]

Low Back Pain. Almost twenty-eight million Americans suffer from back pain. Of those twenty-eight million, 80 percent suffer pains attributable to physical deterioration, which can be reversed with physical exercise.[18] Kraus and Raab have clearly stated the reason why back pain is such a frequent complaint today:

> Since our civilization does not permit the natural response of fight or flight, since we do not have vicarious outlets by heavy exercise, tension is stored up in our muscles. This constant tension shortens muscles and deprives them of elasticity. Once this muscle tightness has reached a sufficient high level, and lack of physical activity has weakened our tense muscles, the stage is set for the first episode of back pain.[19]

Reducing Emotional Tension. Exercise is effective in combating tension. The late Dr. Paul Dudley White, M.D., dean of American cardiologists, stressed this benefit of exercise: "Vigorous leg exercise is the best antidote for nervous and emotional stress that we possess, far better than tranquilizers or sedatives to which, unhappily, so many are addicted today." [20]

Research has been conducted to support this contention. Dr. Herbert deVries, Ph.D., working with a group of men fifty years old and older, discovered that a fifteen-minute walk reduced neuromuscular tension more effectively than a dosage of tranquilizers.[21] Dr. Richard Driscoll, Ph.D., reports that his research shows that a program combining exercise and pleasant thoughts helps to banish anxiety.[22]

Greater Productivity and Job Performance. Working capacity is, of course, linked to endurance and stamina. With conditioning comes a greater capacity to get things done. You are able to do more before feeling fatigued. In short, you have more pep.

Exercise physiologists say that to have more energy you must spend energy—not get more rest. That seemingly paradoxical statement summarizes the theory of "aerobic power." Aerobic power refers to the body's ability to process oxygen.

The beneficial effect of sound exercise on job performance has been widely acknowledged. In one study, Dr. Roy Shepard, M.D., Ph.D., of the University of Toronto's Department of Physiological Hygiene, noted the benefits of exercise in increasing endurance on the job. In studying elderly men and women, he saw that many were unable to work an eight-hour day without suffering fatigue. The introduction of a regular exercise plan to this group led to Dr. Shepard's observation that "through the use of an appropriate training program, it is possible to improve the working capacity by at least 15 percent to 29 percent." [23]

Dr. Victor Linden,[24] of Bergen Trygdleasse, Bergen, Norway, points out that employees with high rates of absenteeism are less physically fit and less active during their leisure time than their co-workers with good performance records.

Other Benefits. Although it is still a speculative area, research is being reported that may indicate that exercise can change personality. In one study, a group of researchers at Purdue University found that people who volunteered for a program of regular physical activity became more self-sufficient.[25] Other possible benefits include an extended period of youthfulness,[26] sounder sleep, and less sexual tension.[27]

THE CHOICE IS YOURS

Consumer Guide® believes it is important that you know all the facts and learn to separate them from the guesswork, the half-truths, and the exaggerated claims. Whether you decide to exercise or not is your decision, one you should make with the help of a competent physician. We can provide you with guidelines on how to select the kind of exercise that will help you be fit for life. If a properly selected program is followed regularly, you will see an increase in your ability to meet a day's stress without undue fatigue, maintain an energy reserve to meet most unforeseen demands, and enjoy life more fully.

We can give the guidelines, but you will have to provide the motivation, time, and proper selection of exercise.

2

WHAT IS
PHYSICAL FITNESS?

RIGHT AT THE START LET'S UNDERSTAND ONE THING: THERE is a good bit of confusion over the term "physical fitness."

To each of us physical fitness may mean something different. For some it is the ability to do thirty push-ups; or it may be the ability to run a mile and a half nonstop or to get through the day without fatigue. Or it may simply mean looking or feeling good. Physicians generally regard fitness as freedom from disease; physiologists examine responses to certain stimuli; and physical educators look for the capacity of human performance. All of these have a place in a full definition of fitness.

In this book, the broadest view will be taken. In our definition, fitness encompasses the basic physical well-being necessary for a full and healthy life. The President's Council on Physical Fitness and Sports has issued a concise statement that sums up pretty nicely what physical fitness is all about: "The ability to carry out daily tasks with vigor and alertness, without undue fatigue, and with ample energy to enjoy leisure-time pursuits and to meet unforeseen emergencies." [1]

THE FOUNDATIONS OF FITNESS

Physical fitness is dependent upon two basic components, which we shall refer to as "organic" and "dynamic" fitness.

Both are necessary ingredients in overall physical fitness, and it is the interaction between the two that determines how fit we are.

By "organic fitness" we mean the characteristics of the particular flesh-and-blood body we each possess, inherited from our parents and affected by aging and perhaps by illness or accident. Here we are speaking of body size, build, and other physical features. This is what we're talking about when we say a person comes from "strong stock" or when we speak of another individual as having certain physical limitations or difficulties. This "organism" is essentially static, and difficult or even impossible to alter. Your organic fitness level determines your potential for overall physical fitness.

"Dynamic fitness" is much more variable. This term is here used to refer to the readiness and capacity of the body for action and movement. It has to do not with the ultimate potential for (or we could say limitations on) action, but with the degree to which this potential is realized.

Imagine a "fitness continuum" with two extremes: the ideal "fit" American on one end and the completely incapacitated (and even degenerating) individual on the other. Obviously, people with heart lesions, metabolic diseases, neurological dysfunction, and other disabilities are not in good health, nor are they fit. At the same time, people who are basically in good health yet are very inactive would also be low on the fitness continuum because they are deficient in dynamic fitness, lacking such characteristics as strength and endurance. Dr. George Sheehan, M.D., says that most Americans are in this latter condition, and he calls it "good health; lousy shape." [2]

Organic and dynamic fitness must both be considered in any evaluation of fitness; neither predominates. For example, you may have inherited a body that could conceivably run a four-minute mile, but smoking, inactivity, stress, and poor diet may result in your being able to walk only a mile in twenty minutes. In other words, your life-style has hampered the development of the important components of fitness—circulo-respiratory endurance. Although you are organically sound, your dynamic fitness is low and your overall fitness suffers greatly.

This works the other way, too. You may have inherited a capacity to run only a six-minute mile, yet daily jogging, no smoking, and good diet permit you to work close to your potential. In that case, your overall fitness would be considered quite good.

On the whole, organic fitness is difficult to alter and represents a "given factor" in our chances for all-around physical fitness. We can't change our height, leg and arm length, or general build. If we have inherited physical handicaps of any kind or have experienced an illness or accident that has left a physical disability, we must operate within certain limits that others may not have to cope with.

Dynamic fitness, on the other hand, can be improved greatly merely by doing something about it. Whatever your stature and biological characteristics, you can advance dramatically on the fitness continuum by getting enough of the right kind of exercise. To a large extent, then, dynamic fitness is the focus of attention in this book.

COMPONENTS OF DYNAMIC FITNESS

Most theorists agree that dynamic fitness consists of five major components: muscular strength, muscular endurance, flexibility, circulo-respiratory endurance, and good body composition.[3] These can all be significantly improved through proper exercise. Which components are developed depends upon the type of exercise selected.

MUSCULAR STRENGTH

Muscular strength is measured by the amount of force that can be exerted by a single contraction of a muscle. A reasonable degree of muscle strength is important for many reasons. It's necessary for such household tasks as carrying out the garbage, lifting groceries, and moving furniture, as well as for coping with emergency situations. Adequate shoulder and back strength is needed to help avoid slouching and to maintain proper support for the back. Strength is also necessary in order to have good skill performance in many types of athletics. Muscular strength is developed with exercise such as weight training, isometrics, isokinetics, or selected calisthenics.

MUSCULAR ENDURANCE

Muscular endurance is measured by the length of time a type of activity can be sustained by particular muscles—that is, how many times a person can repeat an exercise, such as arm circles, push-ups, and sit-ups.

We need muscle endurance to continue in any given activity over a period of time. For example, strength is needed to assume a correct postural position, but muscle endurance is essential in order to maintain that posture throughout the day.

Many jobs require muscle endurance. A typist needs sufficient forearm, shoulder, and back muscle endurance to type all day. A bricklayer needs a high degree of muscle endurance to work continuously. Muscle endurance is needed in order to stand or sit at any job for several hours a day without becoming overly fatigued. Without muscle endurance, a person tires quickly and his or her efficiency suffers, thereby cutting down on productivity.

Muscle endurance is improved through calisthenics, weight training, and aerobic exercises.

FLEXIBILITY

Flexibility is the range of motion possible at the joints. For example, from a sitting position—legs straight out in front— can you touch your toes without bending your knees? If you can't, the muscles, tendons, and ligaments of the lower back and back of the legs are not sufficiently flexible.

Flexibility is necessary in all the major joints of the body to help avoid muscle pulls and strains. Improved flexibility will result in fewer injuries, better performance, and more freedom of movement. Lack of flexibility can contribute to lower back pain and those maddening muscle and joint injuries that occur in adults when they attempt to reach for an object underneath a desk or on top of a shelf.

To improve overall flexibility, you must work separately on each joint or group of joints in the body. Flexibility is improved through slow, stretching exercises, continually repeated over a period of time.

CIRCULO-RESPIRATORY ENDURANCE

Circulo-respiratory endurance consists of the ability of the heart, blood, and blood vessels to transport oxygen to the muscle cells, process the oxygen in those cells, and carry off the resultant waste products. Sometimes this is called "aerobic fitness," "aerobic power," or "cardiovascular fitness."

Many physiologists feel that this is the most important component of physical fitness. It determines how well you can persist in large muscle activities for a sustained period of time. A high level of circulo-respiratory endurance is needed for many daily tasks and to handle the unexpected without placing dangerous stress on the body.

Moreover, there is considerable evidence that activities or

exercises that improve circulo-respiratory endurance may help reduce certain cardiovascular disease risk factors in adults. That is, they may provide what is called "cardio-protective resistance" (help prevent heart attacks, in layman's terms).

With a high degree of circulo-respiratory endurance, fatigue is postponed and work can be carried on for longer periods. Circulo-respiratory endurance is important when participating in most sports.

The best exercises for improving circulo-respiratory endurance or cardiovascular endurance are walking, jogging, swimming, dancing, bicycling, and any activities that are of a continuous, dynamic nature involving large muscle groups of the body.

No one can say yet that these exercises will help you live longer, but we do know that they improve heart health and lessen fatigue, so that you will be more productive while you are alive.

Consumer Guide® is among those who believe that circulo-respiratory endurance is the most important component of dynamic fitness. This type of exercise will slow down fatigue, increase energy, reduce body weight, and reduce several coronary heart disease risk factors. No other component of fitness can make all those claims.

BODY COMPOSITION

Research has shown that many degenerative diseases, including heart disease, diabetes, and arthritis, are related to obesity. It is important to note that the reference is to obesity and not to overweight; they are not synonymous. The distinction is simple: "Properly speaking, an obese person is one who carries around an excessive amount of body fat. An overweight person, on the other hand, simply weighs more than what's recommended on the height/weight tables."[4]

Often the height/weight charts used in approximating

desired weight are erroneous or misleading. These charts overlook the importance of percentage of fat in proper determination of ideal weight. (Percent of fat is determined by the use of underwater weighing equipment and skin-fold calipers; we'll have more on this later.) The ideal percentage of body fat for males is around 12 percent (youth) and 15 percent (adult). For females, it's around 19 percent (youth and adult). The upper limits are 20 percent for a young boy or man, 25 percent for a young girl, and 30 percent for an adult woman. When the percentage of body fat is greater, the person is considered obese, even though the charts indicate that his or her weight is in line with what is "normal."

The best activities for weight control are those already listed as contributing to cardiovascular endurance.

FITNESS: THE KEY TO JOYFUL LIVING

Dynamic fitness is high on the list of prerequisites for health and well-being. There are other important factors—selection of nutritious foods, for example. The body needs good fuel and must be protected from substances that damage and waste its resources. You also need adequate rest, regular physical examinations, appropriate medical care, and good relaxation habits. These factors and others should be combined for a program of overall fitness that will help prevent disease, improve the functioning of your body systems, increase efficiency, and perhaps even lengthen your life expectancy.

Most of us have had the experience of beginning an exercise session feeling run-down and tired and then feeling pleasantly tired but somehow uplifted after the exercise. Whether this better feeling is the result of physiological and psychological changes or a sense of worth because of accomplishing a task and disciplining oneself has not been determined. But it is apparent that people on exercise programs have more pep, vigor, and enthusiasm.[5] Some call it a better outlook on life. Others say they feel better, are more confident, and face the problems of living in a more relaxed manner. They learn to lose themselves in play activities and relax, to experience a "joy of living"; this is perhaps the most important product of fitness.

3

HOW FIT ARE YOU?

MOST PEOPLE KNOW THEY NEED EXERCISE. AND MOST PEOPLE need a lot more exercise than they get. The best way to find out how much exercise you should be getting is to test yourself on the five components of dynamic fitness.

FIRST: A PHYSICAL EXAMINATION

Consumer Guide® recommends a physical checkup before starting an exercise program or engaging in the cardio-respiratory tests described in this chapter. The checkup should include examination of the cardiovascular system, muscles, and joints. Ideally, blood should be analyzed for cholesterol and triglycerides, and blood pressure should be noted. A resting electrocardiogram (EKG) should be performed. (In some instances, as will be discussed, an EKG taken while exercising is strongly recommended.)

Most Americans believe they are in fairly good health and shape. Too often they attack an exercise program with excess vigor that can cause serious problems. Many think they can begin exercising with the same enthusiasm they displayed twenty years earlier in their high school or college days. This is dangerous. An examination is recommended because most of us are less than fully aware of our true physical condition and run the risk of injuring ourselves through an over-zealous approach to exercise.

Dr. Kenneth Cooper's recommendations set forth in the *Journal of the American Medical Association* are worthy of consideration. He suggests the following guidelines:

Under 30: You can start exercising if you've had a checkup within the past year and the doctor found nothing wrong with you.

Between 30 and 39: You should have a checkup within three months before you start exercising. The examination should include an electrocardiogram (EKG) taken at rest.

Between 40 and 59: Same as for the 30–39 group, with one important addition—your doctor should also check your heart by taking an EKG while you are exercising.

Over 59: The same requirements as for the 40–59 age group except that the examination should be performed immediately before embarking on any exercise program.[1]

Once you have medical approval of your plan to begin a program of regular exercise, the next step is to decide what kind of activity fits your needs. This is the time to evaluate yourself in terms of each of the five dynamic fitness components.

CIRCULO-RESPIRATORY ENDURANCE: CAN YOUR SYSTEM TAKE IT?

We've already said that the most important component of fitness is circulo-respiratory endurance. The best way to see how you measure up in this area is to take an "exercise stress test"—a test in which an electrocardiogram is taken while you are exercising.* An EKG performed while resting is not at all the same thing. Think of the difference between testing your car in the garage and testing it on the highway at fifty-five miles an hour.

---

* Listings of laboratories providing stress tests may be obtained by contacting National Fitness Director, National Council of YMCAs, 291 Broadway, New York, NY 10007; National Jogging Association, 1910 K Street, No. 202, Washington, DC 20006; and Fitness Finders, 178 E. Harmony, Spring Arbor, MI 49283.

The Exercise Stress Test. In an exercise stress test, the individual pedals a stationary bicycle (a bicycle ergometer), walks or runs on a motorized treadmill, or climbs a bench step while being monitored by an EKG. The activities are much like those one might engage in as part of an exercise program. Exactly how long the exercises continue depends on the type of test and the physician.

During these tests, the EKG is continuously monitored and blood pressure is observed, to guard against overexertion. At the first sign that the heart is irritated by exercise, the test is stopped. By watching the EKG, blood pressure, and respiration rate, the physician or exercise physiologist can tell whether the patient on the treadmill is working to the limit of capacity.

During some of these tests, the patient also breathes into a one-way valve that enables the physician or physiologist to collect the air exhaled. This air is then analyzed to determine the amount of oxygen the body used during the activity. The oxygen used by the body is usually measured in liters per minute and the measurement refined as milliliters of oxygen per kilogram of total body weight. This measurement represents the person's aerobic capacity—the rate at which oxygen is being used. Although many professional groups (such as the American Medical Association, the American Heart Association, and the American College of Sports Medicine) favor oxygen analysis as a preliminary to exercise plans for previously sedentary Americans, this test is usually not given because of the cost and need for additional personnel.

Some experts, Dr. George Sheehan, M.D., among them, are critical of stress testing. He points out that he is not alone in this opinion:

> Some experts think the exercise stress test is highly restrictive, expensive, and probably an unnecessary precaution (Dr. Gordon Cumming, Canadian cardiologist). And others judge it to be of

no great value even in the diagnosis of coronary disease (Dr. Stephen Epstein, National Heart Institute). Further, when given without a warm-up to presumably healthy people, 70 percent abnormal results are obtained (Dr. Albert Kattus, UCLA). And in apparently normal women, ages fifty to sixty, almost half had abnormal stress tests (Dr. Cumming). If this isn't enough to raise doubts, you should note that European physiologists suggest that much of what we call abnormal is simply excess nervous tone.... Don't forget that laboratory tests are just that: Performed at 70 percent temperature and 40 percent humidity with no wind. Changing meteorological conditions, proximity to meals, presence of tension or excitement all change the demands on our cardiopulmonary and muscular systems.[2]

What does it really prove anyway? The screening of dangerous heart conditions is the most obvious reason for the test. But even if nothing serious turns up, it can be used by the physician, exercise physiologist, and you to better gauge your ability to withstand exercise. It's like filling a drug prescription; the dosage must be correct to do the most good. Too little, and it's not effective; too much can be harmful. The stress test enables the tester to identify the proper dosage—how hard, how long, and how frequently.

As important as laboratory "in motion" testing may be, it is not readily available to all people. Kenneth Cooper observes that "stress-testing everyone is not practical. There are not enough treadmills or physicians to provide all the tests. Furthermore, not all of the people are going to have enough money to take the test."[3]

ALTERNATIVES TO STRESS TESTING

Many researchers have tried to come up with other, simpler ways to test circulo-respiratory endurance. Some are especially interesting because they can be administered at home by nonprofessionals—if close attention is paid to accurate measurement and careful observance of the directions. The advocates of these alternatives also suggest checking with your physician prior to taking the tests.

THE KASCH PULSE RECOVERY TEST.[4] One such test is the Kasch Pulse Recovery Test. This test, developed by Dr. Fred Kasch, Ph.D., of San Diego State University, requires only:

1 / a bench or step exactly twelve inches high (a stack of newspapers securely tied together will work, or two six-inch stair steps)
2 / a clock or watch with a sweep second hand
3 / a friend, to help you with the counting

Don't smoke or engage in any type of physical activity for at least two hours before taking this test.

PROCEDURE:
   To begin, step up onto the bench or step, stand fully erect, then step back down from the bench. Do this for three minutes, at the rate of 24 steps per minute. (That's a full step-up-step-down every 2.5 seconds.) Both feet must step onto the bench and return to the floor each time. The action should be even and relaxed, not jumping or hopping: step up on the bench with your right foot, up with your left foot, return your right foot to the floor, and return your left foot to the floor. This completes one cycle.
   In the unlikely event that you find the test too vigorous, stop, and rate your fitness level "poor."
   When you've done this for 3 minutes, sit down and relax—without talking—for 5 seconds. Then take your pulse rate for 60 seconds.
   To get an accurate pulse count, place the middle three fingers of one hand on the underside of the opposite wrist. If you have difficulty locating your pulse there, try placing the same three fingers on either side of your throat just below the joint of the jaw. Count each "push" or "throb" you feel against your fingertips. (Some people need a little practice in finding the pulse; try it once or twice prior to the test.)

To complete the test and determine your fitness level, locate your pulse rate in Figure 2.

FIGURE 2 / CIRCULO-RESPIRATORY ENDURANCE RATINGS, MEASURED BY PULSE RECOVERY RATE [5]

FITNESS LEVEL	6–12 yrs.		18–26 yrs.		33–57 yrs.	
	BOYS	GIRLS	MEN	WOMEN	MEN	WOMEN
Excellent	73–82	81–92	69–75	76–84	63–76	73–86
Good	83–92	93–104	76–83	85–94	77–90	87–100
Average	93–103	105–118	84–92	95–105	91–106	101–117
Fair	104–113	119–130	93–99	106–116	107–120	118–130
Poor	114–123	131–142	100–106	117–127	121–134	131–144

Note: If your age group is not listed, use the figure in the closest age range.

Obviously, this test is not a substitute for a stress test. But it does give you an idea of where you would fall on an aerobic fitness continuum. The test also allows you to better "prescribe" your exercise dosage.

THE COOPER FIELD TEST (1½-MILE RUN/WALK). There is another, more vigorous test that can be used to estimate aerobic fitness. Acknowledging that the stress test is not always practical, Dr. Kenneth Cooper devised a mile-and-a-half run/walk field test, which has been found to correlate highly with the standardized stress test.[6] The objective is to see how fast you can run a mile and a half. To score in the "good" category, you must cover the mile and a half in about twelve minutes. (The time varies according to age and sex, as seen in Figure 3.)

One very important note: This test is *not to be administered unless you have been on a cardiovascular fitness program for at least three months.* You should be able to jog nonstop for fifteen minutes before you consider taking this test. Begin with a proper warm-up and end with adequate cooling-down

FIGURE 3 / 1.5-MILE RUN TEST
TIME (MINUTES)

MEN

FITNESS CATEGORY	AGE (YEARS)					
	13-19	20-29	30-39	40-49	50-59	60+
Very poor	15:31+	16:01+	16:31+	17:31+	19:01+	20:01+
Poor	12:11-15:30	14:01-16:00	14:44-16:30	15:36-17:30	17:01-19:00	19:01-20:00
Fair	10:49-12:10	12:01-14:00	12:31-14:45	13:01-15:35	14:31-17:00	16:16-19:00
Good	9:41-10:48	10:46-12:00	11:01-12:30	11:31-13:00	12:31-14:30	14:00-16:15
Excellent	8:37-9:40	9:45-10:45	10:00-11:00	10:30-11:30	11:00-12:30	11:15-13:59
Superior	Under 8:37	Under 9:45	Under 10:00	Under 10:30	Under 11:00	Under 11:15

WOMEN

FITNESS CATEGORY	AGE (YEARS)					
	13-19	20-29	30-39	40-49	50-59	60+
Very poor	18:31+	19:01+	19:31+	20:01+	20:31+	21:01+
Poor	18:30-16:55	19:00-18:31	19:30-19:01	20:00-19:31	20:30-20:01	21:00-21:31
Fair	16:54-14:31	18:30-15:55	19:00-16:31	19:30-17:31	20:00-19:01	20:30-19:31
Good	14:30-12:30	15:54-13:31	16:30-14:31	17:30-15:56	19:00-16:31	19:30-17:31
Excellent	12:29-11:50	13:30-12:30	14:30-13:00	15:55-13:45	16:30-14:30	17:30-16:30
Superior	Under 11:50	Under 12:30	Under 13:00	Under 13:45	Under 14:30	Under 16:30

Adapted from K. H. Cooper, *The Aerobics Way.* NY: M. Evans, 1977.

exercises. Also, if you find during the test that you are experiencing any type of extreme fatigue, shortness of breath, lightheadedness, or nausea, *stop immediately.* Do not try to repeat the test until your fitness level has been gradually improved through regular exercise. If you experience chest pain during the test, you should see your family physician.

Consumer Guide® recommends that you have your performance measured via a stress test if at all possible. An alternative is the Kasch Pulse Recovery Test. The mile-and-a-half run/walk is to be done *only* after adequate training; if you question at all your ability to complete this distance (to run a mile and a half), you should put yourself into the "very poor" or "poor" fitness category. Only one assumption is safe: If you haven't been exercising, you are in one of these two categories.

BODY COMPOSITION: "WHO, ME—OBESE?"

As already explained, the terms "overweight" and "obese" are not synonymous. Overweight means too much weight according to the height/weight charts (including muscle, bone, fat, etc., with no distinction made as to the proportions of these various components); obesity means an excessive amount of body *fat* (referring specifically to fat tissue).

An overweight man or woman, for example, may well be within the normal range of "fatness." Or even comparatively lean.

Professional football players provide a good example. A halfback may be six feet tall and weigh 205 pounds—too much, according to the tables. But only 10 percent of his total weight is fat (15 or 16 percent is the ideal percentage for men). How can this be? The football player exercises a lot and is heavily muscled. Much of his weight is muscle tissue. Many athletes are overweight but not obese.

On the other hand, a person can be obese without being

overweight according to the tables. It is possible to weigh just what the tables say you ought to weigh, but still have a total percentage of body fat that is several points over what's desirable and healthy.

Many American males fall into this category. A typical case might be the athlete who weighed about 170 pounds in his senior year and eventually became a sedentary member of the desk set. The muscle tissue in his body is less dense and thus less heavy. All else being equal, he should lose weight. However, as usual with most adult Americans today, there is a corresponding enlargement of the fat cells, which accounts for the weight gain. The lean-to-fat ratio changes, and he becomes obese but not actually overweight.

Yes, one can even be obese and *under*weight! In conducting a series of tests on adult males, Dr. Ancel Keys, the eminent Minnesota physiologist, found that 20 percent of his subjects fell into the "underweight but too fat" category. At the same time, between 20 and 30 percent were overweight but within the normal range of fat distribution. Many were, in fact, extremely lean. One interesting finding: the men who were both obese and overweight led very sedentary lives, while the men who were overweight but not fat engaged in heavy labor.[7]

Obviously, the height/weight tables are not the last word. At best, they are a rough guide to how much a person should weigh. If the height/weight tables are so misleading, how can a person know what weight is best for him or her—whether that person is now obese but not overweight, overweight but not obese, both obese and overweight, or whatever?

HYDROSTATIC WEIGHING. By far the most accurate method yet devised to estimate body composition is hydrostatic weighing, carried out while the subject is immersed in water. The amount of water displaced is recorded, and other measurements—residual lung volume, body weight in and out of water, etc.—are made. From these measurements, the proportion of body fat can be calculated. Hydrostatic weighing requires some elaborate and expensive equipment and is obviously not a do-it-yourself project.

MEASURING SKIN-FOLD THICKNESS. A more practical method is the caliper measurement of skin-fold thickness. The National Center of Health Statistics in Washington points out that "skin folds permit a closer estimate of body fat than do the tables of relative weight. ... Skin folds are becoming established as the easiest and most direct measure of body fat available in the doctor's office, the clinic, or in a large-scale population survey." [8]

In most people under the age of fifty, at least half of the body fat is stored directly underneath the skin. By measuring the thickness of the fold produced when the skin and tissue just under it are firmly grasped, it is possible to get a good idea of how much fat is present. Some of the most common locations at which this measurement is taken include the upper arm at the triceps (back of upper arm), the subscapular region (middle of the back at the shoulder blades), the waistline, the biceps (front of upper arm), and the ilium (waistline right above the hipbone), to mention a few.

The National Health Survey results published in 1970 showed that the average triceps (right arm) skin fold of males is .511 inch and that it thickens with age from .433 inch between ages 18 and 24 years to .55 inch between 24 and 44 years of age. Women's right-arm skin folds consistently were thicker, averaging .866 inch. As young adults, women average .708 inch; in middle age they average .984 inch. Skin-fold thicknesses showing obesity are listed in Figure 4.*

THE PINCH TEST. Calipers are precise and scientific, but you are not conducting a research survey. You don't need a caliper to measure your own skin fold to determine whether you are fat. Simply do the pinch test.

---

* For the consumer, a plastic skin-fold caliper (complete with written norms) is available from Dr. H. Company, P.O. Box 266, Chesterfield, MO 63017. Research models are available from Cambridge Scientific Instruments, Cambridge, MD; H. E. Morse Co., Holland, MI; Quinton Instrument Co., Seattle, WA.

FIGURE 4 / MINIMUM TRICEPS SKIN-FOLD
THICKNESS INDICATING OBESITY
INCHES (MILLIMETERS)

AGE (YEARS)	MALES	FEMALES
5	0.4724 (12)	0.55118 (14)
6	0.4724 (12)	0.59055 (15)
7	0.5118 (13)	0.62992 (16)
8	0.55118 (14)	0.66929 (17)
9	0.59055 (15)	0.70866 (18)
10	0.62992 (16)	0.78740 (10)
11	0.66929 (17)	0.82677 (21)
12	0.70866 (18)	0.86614 (22)
13	0.70866 (18)	0.90551 (23)
14	0.66926 (17)	0.90551 (23)
15	0.62992 (16)	0.94455 (24)
16	0.59055 (15)	0.98425 (25)
17	0.55118 (14)	1.02362 (26)
18	0.59055 (15)	1.06299 (27)
19	0.59055 (15)	1.06299 (27)
20	0.62992 (16)	1.10236 (28)
21	0.66929 (17)	1.10236 (28)
22	0.70866 (18)	1.10236 (28)
23	0.70866 (18)	1.10236 (28)
24	0.74803 (19)	1.10236 (28)
25	0.7874 (20)	1.14173 (29)
26	0.7874 (20)	1.14173 (29)
27	0.82677 (21)	1.14173 (29)
28	0.86614 (22)	1.14173 (29)
29	0.86614 (22)	1.14173 (29)
30–50	0.90551 (23)	1.1811 (30)

From: C. C. Seltzer and J. Mayer, "A Simple Criterion of Obesity," *Postgraduate Medicine*, 83, 2 (1965), A-101.

Gently pinch the skin at the triceps of one upper arm (at the back), midway between the shoulder and elbow (with the thumb and forefinger of the other hand). Ideally, the skin fold should be between one quarter and one half of an inch. If you can grasp more than one inch, you can probably conclude you are sliding into the obese range.

CHEST/WAIST MEASUREMENT. There is another homespun way to tell if you are fat. Stand with shoulders pulled back and maximum chest expansion. Measure the circumference of your chest just beneath your armpits. Be certain that your tape measure is flat and level. Then measure your waist (at the navel), with your stomach in a relaxed position—not sucked in or forced out. For men the chest should be five inches greater in circumference than the waist; for women the difference should be ten inches.

THE WEIGHT GAIN TEST. Another test is simply to recall what you weighed when you were twenty-one if you are a woman, or twenty-five if you are a man. If memory fails, you can dig out old medical records. You can assume that each pound gained since that time represents an accumulation of fat.

THE MIRROR TEST. The quickest, easiest way to find out if you are too fat is to get undressed and stand in front of a full-length mirror. Be critical. Do you like what you see? Have your body contours changed? If you look fat, you can reasonably conclude that you are fat. If you sag where you don't want to sag, if you can "pinch an inch" of fat on your body, if your waist protrudes, you probably are moving into the obese range, or you are already there.

FLEXIBILITY: CAN YOU MOVE?

Flexibility refers to the range of motion possible at a joint or series of joints.

It is inaccurate to speak of a person as flexible or inflexible; flexibility is specific to each particular joint or combination of joints. It is possible to be flexible in the shoulder area and yet have very poor low back flexibility. Most people tend to lack flexibility in the back of the thigh (hamstring), low back, neck, and chest.

At some joints the degree of movement is very definitely limited by the bone structure itself or by the bulk of the muscles between the joints. Flexion and extension at the knee joint is an example. Extension (straightening or increasing the angle of the joint) is definitely limited by the joint structure, and flexion (bending or decreasing the angle of the joint) by the size of the thigh and calf muscles. Some joints (the ankle, hip, and shoulder, for example) have flexibility limits set primarily by the ease and degree to which the muscles, connective tissue (tendons and ligaments), and skin can be stretched.

Our sedentary living habits are the major contributors to loss of flexibility. Inactivity causes muscles and connective tissue to lose elasticity. An increase in body fat, which is definitely related to inactivity, also contributes to decreased flexibility.[9]

Poor flexibility can result in poor body movement—whether walking, running, sitting, or standing. It also contributes to joint and muscle pain and greater likelihood of injury to muscles, tendons, and ligaments.

Because flexibility is specific to each joint, there is no general test that indicates total body flexibility fitness. Each joint must be tested separately.

THE SITTING TOE TOUCH. The 1975 *Official YMCA Physical Fitness Handbook* outlines a flexibility test for two major areas of the body--low back and back of the thigh.[10] These particular areas are significant because low back pain is such a disabling and frequent condition in the United States.

To perform this test you will need a yardstick and adhesive tape.

PROCEDURE:
Warm up with some stretching before the test.

Sit on the floor with legs extended and heels about 5 inches apart.

With a strip of adhesive tape, mark the place where the heels touch the floor. The heels are to touch the near edge of the tape.

Place the yardstick on the floor between and parallel to the legs so that the fifteen-inch mark touches the near edge of the taped heel line (with beginning of yardstick toward you).

Slowly reach with both hands as far forward as possible. Touch the fingertips to the yardstick and hold this position momentarily. The yardstick shows the distance reached. *Do not attempt to add length by jerking forward.*

Do this three times, recording the distance in inches each time. Circle your best score.

Your flexibility rating is determined by finding your score in Figure 5.

FIGURE 5 / LOW BACK AND HAMSTRING FLEXIBILITY RATINGS, MEASURED BY SITTING TOE TOUCH DISTANCE [11]

RATING	MEN	WOMEN
Excellent	22–23 inches	24–27 inches
Good	20–21 inches	21-23 inches
Average	14–19 inches	16–20 inches
Fair	12–13 inches	13–16 inches
Poor	0–11 inches	0–12 inches

MUSCULAR STRENGTH: ARE YOU STRONG ENOUGH?

Muscular strength refers to the measurement of maximum strength in a single muscular contraction. The length of time of the contraction is not a factor.

To test this component of physical fitness, it is necessary to decide which muscles are going to be tested for strength. If the measuring of biceps muscle strength, for example, is a goal, it is necessary to measure the amount of weight that can be lifted with the arms at one time. Leg strength might be measured by how high an individual can jump. The test used most frequently to determine strength is the grip-strength test. Researchers have found that this test correlates very highly with overall body strength.[12]

A hand-grip dynamometer or manuometer is necessary for this test. This instrument is held in the hand and squeezed as tightly as possible. The dynamometer records in pounds or kilograms the strength of the subject's grip.

THE MODIFIED KRAUS-WEBER TEST. It is possible to measure *minimum* muscular strength at home. The following tests are modifications of a program proposed by Dr. Hans Kraus.[13] Each of the six is scored simply as "pass" or "fail."

PROCEDURE:

Test No. 1: Strength of the abdominal and psoas (loin) muscles. Lie on back, hands behind your neck; the examiner holds your feet down. Perform one sit-up.

Test No. 2: Strength of the abdominal muscles without the help of the psoas. Begin in the position used for Test No. 1. Bending your knees, draw the heels close to the buttocks. In this position, perform one sit-up.

Test No. 3: Strength of the psoas and lower abdominal muscles. Begin in the position used for Test No. 1. Lift your legs, fully extended, until the heels are ten inches off the table or floor. Hold this position for ten seconds.

Test No. 4: Strength of the upper back muscles. Lie face down with a pillow under your hips and lower abdomen, hands behind your neck; the examiner holds your feet down. Raise your chest, head, and shoulders and hold them off the table or floor for ten seconds.

Test No. 5: Strength of lower back. Begin in the position used for Test No. 4; the examiner holds your upper back down. Raise your legs off the table or floor, with knees straight, and hold this position for ten seconds.

Test No. 6: Push-up. Lie face down on table or floor with the feet together, elbows bent, hands under your shoulders, palm down. With body straight, push your body off the floor by straightening your arms; return to the starting position. Perform one push-up.

This test simply measures minimum muscular strength. Dr. Kraus states that a failure to pass any one of these tests is an indication of a strength level so low that a person's entire body health is endangered.

MUSCLE ENDURANCE: SIT-UPS

Good muscle endurance permits you to perform a specific task for a length of time without muscle fatigue.

Muscular endurance, like muscular strength, is difficult to measure because there are so many different muscles and muscle groups. Most experts feel, however, that the sit-up is fairly representative of general muscular endurance.[14] It involves one of the most important muscle groups for adults.

PROCEDURE:

Lie flat on back, with hands on thighs and feet slipped under a bed, couch, or heavy chair. Raise the head, then the shoulders and upper trunk, in an upward curl, sliding hands forward until fingertips just touch the kneecaps. Return to flat position.

Your muscle endurance rating is determined by finding your score on the Figure 6 chart.

FIGURE 6 / MUSCULAR ENDURANCE RATING, MEASURED IN SIT-UPS [15]

RATING	MEN	WOMEN
Excellent	50+	50+
Good	40–49	35–49
Average	25–39	22–34
Fair	15–24	12–21
Poor	Less than 14	Less than 12

SUMMING UP: HOW FIT ARE YOU?

Now you have it in a nutshell—or you will when you put it all down in one place and take a look. Summarize your ratings in the following chart.

Now you know where you stand. If you circled "yes" for any of these test items, you need work in that area. In the following chapters, we'll discuss what you can do to improve your performance. Just keep a slip of paper noting your key problem areas. (Remember, the most important are circulo-respiratory endurance, body composition, and flexibility.)

FIGURE 7 / YOUR FITNESS STATUS

	RATING	NEED TO IMPROVE? (CIRCLE ONE)
CIRCULO-RESPIRATORY ENDURANCE (The ratings should be "good" or better.)		
Stress test	_____	Yes No
Kasch Pulse Recovery Test	_____	Yes No
1½-mile run/walk	_____	Yes No
BODY COMPOSITION		
Percent fat (The goal is 15% for men, 19% for women.)	_____	Yes No
Skin-fold thickness	_____	Yes No
Chest/Waist Measurement (Chest must be 5 to 10 inches greater than waist for good score.)	_____	Yes No

Weight-gain Test (If you
have gained more than
5 pounds, you need to
improve) _____ Yes No
Pinch test _____ Yes No
Mirror test _____ Yes No

FLEXIBILITY
Sitting toe touch (The
rating should be
"good" or better.) _____ Yes No

MUSCLE STRENGTH
Modified Kraus-Weber
Test (This test is passed
only if *all six* parts are
passed.) _____ Yes No
#1 abdominal plus
psoas muscles _____
#2 abdominal
without psoas
muscles _____
#3 psoas and lower
abdominal
muscles _____
#4 upper back
muscles _____
#5 lower back _____
#6 push-ups _____

MUSCLE ENDURANCE
Sit-ups (The rating should
be "good" or better.) _____ Yes No

4

HOW MUCH
AND WHAT KIND
OF EXERCISE?

A DOCTOR PRESCRIBING MEDICATION IS CAREFUL ABOUT dosage. He considers the weight and size of the patient, the age, the severity of the ailment, possible side effects, and the patient's health status (does he or she have cardiovascular disease, diabetes, a kidney ailment?). Even how long and how often the medication is to be given are matters of careful consideration.

It should be the same with exercise. "Get some more exercise" is not good advice. Exercise physiologists talk about the "pharmacopoeia" of exercise—the prescription of exercise. They say that you and your doctor must consider the mode (type), intensity (how hard), duration (how long), and frequency (how often).[1]

CIRCULO-RESPIRATORY ENDURANCE AND
BODY COMPOSITION

As we've said before, the two most important components of fitness are circulo-respiratory endurance and body composition (proportion of fat tissue). We can consider them together here because there is a great deal of overlap in the exercise best suited to each.

WHAT KIND OF ACTIVITY?

If the goal of an exercise program is to increase circulorespiratory endurance and improve body composition (burn calories), the exercise may be any that involves large muscle masses and is performed continuously for a significant period of time. It must be vigorous enough to engage your whole body.

During such exercise your heart beats faster, your breathing becomes deeper, and your blood vessels expand and open up to carry oxygen and blood to the working muscles. In short, it places a demand on your heart, blood vessels, lungs, and muscles. A regular program of such exercise improves your body's ability to consume, transport, and utilize oxygen; in other words, such exercise is "aerobic."

The most popular activities involving large muscle masses throughout the body are walking, jogging, cycling, and swimming. You may also select dancing, rope skipping, running in place, racket sports, soccer, basketball, and the like, as long as the activity is carried out continuously.

This second element—that the exercise be steady and continuous over a period of time—is crucial:

> Aerobic exercise is the type which steadily supplies enough oxygen to the exercising muscles for as long as the exercise is continued. Any rhythmic, repetitive dynamic activity which can be continued for two or more minutes, without huffing and puffing afterwards, is probably aerobic.[2]

These exercises should not be confused with some others that may be strenuous but are not rhythmic and steady. A jogger, bicyclist, or swimmer is engaging in a "pay as you go" type of exercise. In other words, enough oxygen is taken in to meet the demands of the exercise. A person running very fast or sprinting, however, is not involved in aerobic activity; the sprinter cannot keep up that pace.

Another exercise that does *not* permit sustained activity is weight lifting. Weight lifting may be vigorous and do wonders for the skeletal muscles of your body, but it does very little for your most important muscle—the heart. The problem here is that the activity is not sustained. When lifting, the body is exercising vigorously, but you must rest after such intense effort. Here the drawback is the intermittent pattern of the lifting.

The American Heart Association Committee on Exercise points out the disadvantages of this type of sport:

> Activities requiring effort against heavy resistance such as weight lifting at near-maximum exertion and isometric exercises (tensing one set of muscles against another or against an immovable object) do little to improve cardiovascular function, and are not recommended since they provoke an excessive, possibly dangerous pressor [blood pressure] response.[3]

Such popular activities as bowling and golf are also not effective as aerobic exercise because in these, too, the action is not sustained.

Golf, for example, may help a person relieve tension (if it does not create it!) and thereby provide pleasure. But it contributes practically nothing to conditioning the cardiovascular system. To get any cardiovascular benefit, you would have to carry your clubs, walk briskly between holes (four or more miles per hour), hit the ball with little delay, and play in a twosome or less. (The average person covers the golf course at a rate of about one mile per hour.)

Bowling presents the same problem. The action is intermittent. While you are delivering the ball, the effort is somewhat intense, but then you return to your seat and rest until it is your turn again.

Even calisthenics may be insufficient. Most calisthenics programs tell you to do push-ups, rest, do sit-ups, rest, etc. The "rest" is the problem. For exercise to be effective in conditioning the heart and lungs and burning calories, you must keep moving.

Fortunately, some calisthenics programs can be adapted for use in aerobic conditioning. The idea is to keep moving from one exercise to another, smoothly and without pause. You might try doing your running in place in the kitchen and your knee-bends in the living room if you are getting bored with the scenery. The point is to move and keep moving.[4]

The key words, then, in describing the type of exercise to be selected for cardiovascular and body composition condition are "continual," "rhythmic" and "whole body." Exercises that consist of erratic stopping and starting are indeed exercises and may serve other purposes, but they do little to develop aerobic endurance. And they are among the less effective calorie users.

HOW HARD SHOULD YOU EXERCISE?

The intensity of an exercise refers to the amount of exertion put into the activity—how hard are you working?

A certain level of vigor in exercise is necessary to condition the heart, blood, blood vessels, and muscles. And, of course, the number of calories used in any given exercise is directly related to its intensity.

Finding the right intensity is not simple. The exertion level must be neither too low nor excessive. Authorities in this field have come up with a way to determine the ideal intensity for aerobic exercise. Dr. Lenore Zohman, M.D., Director of Cardiopulmonary Rehabilitation at Montefiore Hospital in New York City, describes this "ideal" exertion level:

There is a target zone in which there is enough activity to achieve fitness, but not too much to exceed safe limits. The name of the game is finding your target zone. Each individual's target zone is between 60 percent and 80 percent of his own maximal aerobic power.[5]

Below 60 percent of capacity, you achieve little fitness benefit unless you participate for an extended period of time (or you were extremely unfit to begin with). Above 80 percent, the added benefit is negligible, as Zohman explains:

> The concept of maximal aerobic power (sometimes called maximal aerobic capacity or maximal oxygen intake) is merely the technical description of the fact that there is a point for each of us where, despite our best efforts, the heart and circulation cannot deliver any more oxygen to the tissues and we cannot exercise much longer or harder without approaching exhaustion.
>
> At this point, the lungs are making oxygen available to the bloodstream but that oxygen cannot be transported by the blood to the muscles fast enough to create enough energy for exercise.

Dr. Zohman's next statement is most interesting: "Almost simultaneously with reaching this limitation of oxygen supply, the heart becomes unable to beat any faster." [6]

This close relationship between maximal aerobic power and maximal attainable heart rate can be the basis for determining the proper intensity for your exercise. In nearly all normal individuals, activity sustained at 60 percent to 80 percent of maximal aerobic power will be accompanied by a heartbeat that is 70 percent to 85 percent of his or her maximal attainable heart rate. This is a very useful fact, as Dr. Zohman explains:

> Because we are able to count our own heart rates, but cannot easily determine our own aerobic power, the heart rate target zone gives us a means of regulating our own exercise performance. If you cannot have your actual maximal heart rate measured, you could assume you are "average" and look up your maximal and target zone heart rate.[7]

But it isn't difficult to measure heart rate; you do this by taking your pulse immediately after strenuous exercise.

Follow the directions carefully and compare your rate to the levels recommended in Figure 8.

FIGURE 8 / DETERMINING TARGET HEART RATE
FOR AEROBIC EXERCISE

The easiest places to count your pulse or heart rate are the radial artery in the wrist and the carotid artery in the neck. For the wrist, turn your palm up and move the second, third and fourth fingers of the other hand along the thumb side of your wrist until you feel a steady pulsation. Or run the same three fingers along your neck about an inch below the curve of the jawbone until you locate the pulse. (Practice finding your pulse a few times before beginning exercise.)

After strenuous exercise, your heart rate drops off rapidly. For this reason, the pulse must be measured immediately upon ending the exercise, and the count should last only fifteen seconds. Using a stopwatch or a clock with a sweep second hand, count the number of beats in fifteen seconds. Then multiply by four for the beats per minute.

AGE	TARGET HEART RATE
20	140 to 170 beats per minute
30	130 to 160 beats per minute
40	125 to 150 beats per minute
50	115 to 140 beats per minute
60	105 to 130 beats per minute

As you can see in the table, the ideal exercise intensity for most people (for aerobic conditioning) occurs at a level accompanied by a rate somewhere between 115 and 170 beats per minute. The specific rate for you depends upon your age. If you are jogging, for example, you could check your pulse immediately after covering one mile. If it is in the target area, that is the proper speed for you. If it is too high, you had better jog at a slower pace, or walk.

HOW LONG?

The next important consideration in planning exercise for circulo-respiratory and body composition improvement is the length of time an exercise is to be continued. This time is usually measured in minutes.

There is a good bit of controversy over how long a person should exercise. To cite two extremes, Dr. Laurence E. Morehouse, Ph.D., suggests ten minutes, three times a week;[8] while Dr. Thomas Bassler, M.D., suggests sixty minutes, six times a week.[9] Dr. Morehouse points to his own research to support his contention.[10] Most researchers, however, indicate that, for ten minutes of activity to have a training effect, the intensity of exercise would have to be too severe for most people.

Dr. Bassler's research is also subject to criticism. He has done autopsies on people who had been joggers or runners and also examined reports from around the world on people who were joggers and died of a heart attack. His conclusion is that there has been no documented heart attack death of a person who was able to complete a marathon (twenty-six miles), was a nonsmoker, and trained at least six miles a day, six days a week.[11] This statement at best is quite speculative.

Somewhere between these extremes lies the optimal amount of exercise for most Americans. Part of the confusion stems from failing to take intensity into account when comparing these estimates. The duration of an activity is inversely related to its intensity. That is, the more intense the activity, the shorter the duration should be; or the less intense, the longer the duration. The American College of Sports Medicine reports that "significant cardiovascular improvements have been obtained with exercise sessions of five to ten minutes' duration with an intensity of more than 90 percent of functional capacity." [12] The College also notes, however, that this high intensity/short duration exercise is not recommended for most participants. Better and safer results are obtained with lower intensities and longer durations.

Another reason for the controversy over duration is lack of agreement on the objectives of a fitness program. If you want to make minimum fitness improvements, ten minutes of exercise might possibly produce some changes. It might enable you to score "satisfactory" on a fitness test. But there are other considerations: It would not necessarily mean that you would achieve a reduction in coronary heart disease risk factors, for example. Experts [13] are very critical of Morehouse's thesis, but more on this later. On the other hand, Dr. Bassler states that "possible insurance" against coronary heart disease requires sixty minutes of running-type exercise daily.[14] Experts [15] have also been very critical of Bassler's research and conclusions. *Consumer Guide*® believes that fifteen to thirty minutes of target-zone exercise is the minimum, yet adequate, amount of time for desirable fitness benefits.

It's easy to get a rough estimate of the amount of exercise you need to achieve weight control. First, estimate your caloric imbalance. (A quick way to think of how many pounds you struggle with each year: If 5 pounds is your problem, you are out of balance by 50 calories per day; 10 pounds—100 calories; 15 pounds—150 calories, etc. Simply add a zero to the number of pounds and this will give you the approximate number of calories you are out of balance.[16])

For every hundred calories you are out of balance, you will need eight to twelve minutes of exercise in the target zone.

HOW OFTEN SHOULD YOU EXERCISE?

Most exercise physiologists believe that circulo-respiratory fitness is best improved and maintained by vigorous exercise five times a week.[17] But there is convincing evidence that comparable benefits can be obtained by participating in organized training programs of approximately thirty minutes three times a week.[18] This view is shared by Dr. Lenore Zohman: "Dynamic, aerobic exercise must be carried out three times weekly with no more than two days elapsing between workouts or gains will begin to be lost." [19] And the American Heart Association concurs: "A daily exercise routine is desirable but cardiovascular fitness may be enhanced by properly regulated sessions at least three days a week." [20]

The case may be different for body composition. Some studies conclude that exercising three days per week is not enough to effect change in body composition. Dr. Michael Pollock, Ph.D., director of the Institute of Aerobic Research, found that four days a week is effective.[21] This observation was supported by recent research that showed that four-day-a-week exercise was far superior to two-day-a-week in altering body composition.[22]

SUMMARY OF HOW LONG, HARD, AND OFTEN

Learn to "listen" to your body. If it's telling you the time has come for more vigorous exercise, then respond accordingly. For example, at first a brisk walk or doubles tennis may keep your heart in the 70 percent range. But as you become more efficient (more fit), a game of tennis singles or even jogging may become necessary to keep the heart in the 70 percent range.

Let's not forget one precaution: you want to be careful that you do not become excessively winded. (You should be able to hold a conversation with somebody next to you.)

So the prescription for improved circulo-respiratory fitness and body composition is relatively simple for most people: fifteen to thirty minutes of target-range exercise three or four times a week, preceded by a five- to ten-minute warm-up and concluded by a five- to ten-minute cool-down.

This prescription will put you well on the road to overall fitness, but it is not the whole story. The other components of fitness—flexibility, muscle strength, and muscle endurance— also demand some attention.

FLEXIBILITY

Good flexibility contributes much to overall fitness: it permits graceful movement and decreases the chances of injury.

Flexibility—the range of motion possible at a joint or a series of joints—tends to be specific to a particular joint or part of the body. In order to improve flexibility, then, the exercise must also be specific to a joint.

Flexibility exercise is most often needed in the back of the legs (hamstrings), low back, front of the hip, neck, chest, and shoulder. To improve flexibility, you must do some basic exercises that affect the large muscle groups in these areas.

The key element in flexibility exercise is slow, sustained stretching:

> The type of stretching movement used in a flexibility program is very important. ... If you use fast, jerky, bouncy movements, this causes the muscle you are attempting to stretch to contract at the same time. This reduces the effectiveness of your stretching and often causes muscle soreness.
>
> By using a slow, sustained stretch, the receptors [nerve endings] cause the muscle to relax and lengthen and thus aid in

obtaining increased flexibility. Much of the muscle soreness is prevented or alleviated by this type of movement.[23]

You should not become winded during flexibility training. Movement is slow, which means intensity is low.

FREQUENCY AND DURATION

The frequency with which you should do these stretching exercises has not been firmly established. The length of time you spend depends partly, of course, upon how active or inactive you are.

Some current research suggests that alternate-day or every-day participation is best. For most people, five to six minutes of stretching before and after target-zone exercise on a daily or alternate-day basis would be about right.[24]

WHEN: THE WARM-UP

A good way to include stretching and joint exercise in your regular exercise program is to use stretching for your warm-up.

The warm-up is preparation for vigorous exercise by beginning mild exercise and gradually increasing intensity. This allows the heart, lungs, muscles, joints, etc., to adapt to the increasing activity.

Getting people quickly out of a sedentary state into vigorous exercise is not sound. A few minutes should be spent on warm-up exercises. Proper warm-up increases the elasticity of the muscles and tendons, helps prevent strains, and begins to open up pathways to the muscles being used. It also raises the temperature of the muscles and helps to facilitate biochemical reactions that supply energy to the muscle tissues.[25]

Exactly how much warm-up is necessary depends on the individual, but a good general rule is to allow five to ten minutes for warm-up. This warm-up phase is an excellent time to work on flexibility. During the warm-up, your target-zone heart rate should be approached but not exceeded.

THE COOL-DOWN

Flexibility exercise is also a good choice for the cool-down period following vigorous exercise. The cool-down is, in fact, the warm-up in reverse. Instead of preparing your body for activity, the idea is to prepare it to return to its normal working level.

During exercise, your heart pumps blood at a fast rate in order to supply the active muscles with more oxygen and life-sustaining nutrients. Blood is pushed into these muscles by the forceful contractions of your heart, but there is no similar force removing the blood from the muscles and returning it to the heart. Instead, blood is pushed (squeezed) out of the veins and back to the heart by the pressure of the exercising muscles. To aid this process, the veins have one-way valves which ensure that the blood will move in only one direction—toward the heart.

When you suddenly stop exercising, your heart continues its rapid pumping rate for a time. But the muscles are no longer active, and there is, therefore, less pressure on the nearby veins. An excess amount of blood may temporarily collect in the muscles and veins, resulting in light-headedness or chills.

A cooling-down period of less intense exercise allows your heart to slow down gradually. The circulatory system can adapt gradually to the lesser demands of normal activity.

Consumer Guide® recommends that all exercise programs be preceded with a warm-up of at least five to ten minutes and a tapering-off of five to ten minutes. Anything less than that is dangerous and strongly disapproved.

MUSCLE ENDURANCE AND STRENGTH

Many people find that their muscle strength and endurance is adequate. Most would also find that these components will be improved in any aerobic fitness program. However, if you find that you are unable to pass the Kraus-Weber Test described earlier, experience poor strength in your favorite sport, or have a good bit of local muscle fatigue while engaging in your exercises, you should read this next section carefully.

Muscle strength refers to the maximum strength in a single contraction of a particular muscle or muscle group for a short period of time. Muscle endurance, on the other hand, is the ability to sustain work for a longer period of time. You may have a great deal of strength and yet have very little endurance, or vice versa.

Dr. L. E. Morehouse, Ph.D., gives this illustration:

> If we took a prize fighter who had trained for pure strength and put him in the ring with one who had trained for pure endurance, the latter would have to stay out of the former's way for a couple of rounds, but thereafter he would be able to carry the fight. The fighter who trained for pure strength would have to land his knockout blow in the first or second round. After that, he would be finished.[26]

To develop muscle endurance you must adopt the "overload" principle: the muscles should be repeatedly and regularly stimulated by greater than normal exercise. In muscle endurance training, the emphasis is placed on high repetition and low resistance; in other words, the exercise is performed many times and the work load is relatively light. The resistance, however, cannot be so low that there is no appreciable overload.

Specifically, muscle endurance exercises should be repeated at a rate of about thirty per minute. You should reach exhaustion in that period of time. If you are exhausted before that, the load is too heavy, and you are developing more strength than endurance. If, on the other hand, you are able to exercise longer than a minute or so, the work load is too easy, and you are not really overloading the muscles. It is sufficient to work on muscle endurance by exercising three to four times a week or every other day.

Calisthenics can be used very effectively to improve muscle endurance. Most circulo-respiratory exercise programs also contribute something to muscle endurance.

Developing muscle strength also is based on the overload principle, but with reversed emphasis. Instead of low resistance and high repetition, the exercise should feature high resistance and fewer repetitions. That means that your goal is no longer thirty repetitions per minute; the activity should be so strenuous that you become exhausted after six or eight repetitions. There is an interplay between these components. And many times when you are working on muscle endurance you are also developing muscle strength.

For most people, muscle endurance problems seem to occur in the upper and middle third of the body. To be complete, therefore, any exercise program should include some abdominal exercises such as sit-ups, v-seats, and up-oars to condition the abdominal muscles, plus exercises that activate the shoulder and arm muscles.

Weight training (which is simply weight lifting with emphasis on exercise rather than competition) is considered the fastest and best method for improving strength. One of the reasons for this is that it allows for a great deal of precision in controlling the exercise load and specifying the muscles being worked on. Weight training also lends itself easily to flexibility work. The average person, however, need not use weights. Calisthenics will be adequate. Dr. David Clarke, Ph.D., at the University of Maryland says that for the average person calisthenics will be sufficient to develop adequate muscle strength. Dr. Richard Berger, Ph.D., of

Temple University said that some exercises provide enough resistance to develop strength while others do not. Only if the exercise can be performed maximally for about thirty repetitions or less is it a strength and muscle developer. If more than thirty repetitions are possible, the exercise develops more muscular endurance than strength.

Consumer Guide® recommends calisthenics and weight training as unsurpassed in developing and maintaining both muscle endurance and muscle strength. (Calisthenics alone is usually sufficient for these purposes.)

IN SUMMARY

Circulo-respiratory fitness is the most important component of overall fitness. This cannot be neglected. Body composition is next, followed closely by flexibility. Muscle strength and endurance are somewhat lower on the priority scale but should not be overlooked.

If all you have is thirty minutes to exercise, you should select a program of about five minutes' warm-up, twenty minutes' target-rate exercise, and approximately five minutes' tapering off. If you have more time, it is advisable to incorporate some muscle endurance or muscle strength work. (The muscle strength and endurance exercises may be incorporated into the workout right after the warm-up or before the tapering off.) These workouts should be performed three or four times a week, or every other day.

In this book, each exercise program will be evaluated in terms of its contribution to physical fitness. Your responsibility, however, extends one step further: you have to find a program that meets your fitness needs *and* is appealing to you—one you will stay with.

5

BEYOND GOOD INTENTIONS: CHOOSING AN EXERCISE PLAN YOU WON'T DROP

If you've read thoughtfully up to this point, you are no doubt convinced that your body needs exercise. You probably know just what you want out of a fitness program. You've taken a good look at your own level of fitness in each of the five fitness components and decided where you most need work. You're ready to get started and need only to select the exercises for your personal plan.

If you are like most people, you are afraid your good intentions will last only about two or three weeks. We all know about good intentions. In exercise, just like anything else, they aren't enough to keep us going. Many people select an activity that does not fit their current health status, their physique, life-style, or age. Consequently, they soon drop out because of lack of progress, difficulty, and inconvenience.

In an earlier chapter we provided you with some important guidelines regarding the type, vigor, duration, and frequency of exercise best suited to developing fitness. But that is not the whole story. Your interests, health status, body type, age, sex, and time availability are also important factors.

INTEREST

Probably the most important consideration of all—in terms of making a long-range commitment to exercise—is enjoyment. Select an activity you enjoy. There is no question about it: exercising on a regular basis takes discipline. If you select exercises you like, the chances are a lot better that you will stick to the program. This point is obvious, but too often neglected.

Be careful, however, to base your choice on interest, not fad. Don't select an activity because it's "the thing to do." Jogging is very popular these days, and some people who have no real interest in the sport get involved just because all their neighbors are doing it (it's fashionable).

Exercise should never be drudgery, and it never will be if you plan your program carefully. Keep in mind these Nine Principles of Fitness Exercise.

THE PLEASURE PRINCIPLE

Choose activities you enjoy. Too many people base a program on what they think is "good for them" or "good because it hurts." Many follow extremely strict regimens that are doomed to failure. Exercise, for them, is a test of willpower. But that approach will not and does not work for most Americans. Most of us aren't masochists; we're hedonists. We do things for pleasure.

In *Rating the Exercises* we will try to give you enough options for you to find a way to get and remain fit *and* enjoy doing it. The point is that you probably needn't do anything that's going to be a chore or a bore. If you loathe a particular activity, stay away from it. If jogging is not your thing, or getting to the tennis courts is a hassle, don't bother. And don't *feel guilty* about the fact that you don't like to jog or to play tennis. You're unique and have your own interests and abilities. Dr. Kenneth Cooper acknowledges over 28 activities as aerobic (and there are probably quite a few more that he hasn't thought of).

THE TIME PRINCIPLE

The key to sticking to a program is a time commitment. You must be willing to set aside a certain period of time each or every other day. Be specific, and know yourself. Are you an early morning person, a noon person, or an evening person? If morning is your time, that may be the best time for you to exercise. If you function better later in the day, that may be best. At first a little experimenting may be necessary to find out what works best for you.

Whatever you do, don't worry about taking the time. You're doing something positive for your body, and it will make you feel better, more productive, and more alive. And remember, we are asking a time commitment of about 1 percent to 2 percent of your time.

THE SPOUSE PRINCIPLE

Your spouse has to be on your side. Research has shown that your chances of sticking with a program are better if your spouse approves and encourages you.

THE GROUP PRINCIPLE

If you fear your motivation is weak, join a good exercise group or get a few friends to exercise with you. "Working out with a friend gives you the advantage of companionship and having somebody to encourage you when you feel like quitting. This is especially important for joggers. You will jog more if you have someone to talk to and to keep you company." [1]

THE GOAL PRINCIPLE

Goals are important in life, and they're important in a fitness program, too. They give you something specific to work toward and a standard by which to measure your progress. When you are setting a goal, avoid vague generalizations: "I want to get in shape," or "I want to lose weight." Instead, set both a specific long-term goal and some short-terms goals.

For example, if you want to lose weight, determine your best weight and give yourself a long-term goal of perhaps six months or a year. Your short-term goal may be three pounds by the end of the first month.

Perhaps a good rule of thumb is to add just a little bit extra to what you think you are able to do for the short-term goals. That way, you will be motivated to do a little extra work toward your long-term goal.

THE PROGRESS PRINCIPLE

A progress chart lets you compete with yourself. It also tells you and anyone else who looks at the chart how well you are doing on your program. The chart doesn't have to be complicated. The simplest method would be to mark the information on a calendar. Another would be to record mileage jogged or bicycled on a map.

THE SUCCESS PRINCIPLE

Whenever you feel on the verge of quitting, try this. Recall your first workout at the beginning of your fitness program (it may have been running only a half-mile or engaging in twenty minutes of light calisthenics); repeat this exercise. You'll be amazed at how easy it is. This can be just the inspiration you need to return to your exercise program the next day.

THE VARIETY PRINCIPLE

Don't be afraid to put variety into your workout. If you happen to be traveling and you're a jogger, you may find running in the streets of Dallas, Jacksonville, and Charlotte most stimulating. As you run, look around at your surroundings. If you find that your bicycling route is getting you down, try a new area, or try another sport for a while.

BEHAVIOR CHANGE PRINCIPLE

Eliminate habits that have contributed to your sedentary life-style. Replace them with habits more suitable to your goal of increased activity. Such changes as meeting new and active friends, learning a new sport, and reducing TV time are important.

One of the best things you can do is to get your children started in fitness activities that will keep them active for their entire life. To do that, start early. Active children learn more because they experience more body positions and movements. Their brains and nervous systems are stimulated, which enhances their learning experiences. Keeping a child in a crib or playpen all day is a grave injustice. They need activity and explorative movement—not restraint. When they get older, teach them the sports they can use for a lifetime—walking, jogging, cross-country skiing, or bicycling.

A child learns by observing. If parents watch television all evening, ride to the store when they could walk, and adopt sedentary activities as "recreation," their children will learn to be inactive.

HEALTH STATUS

Obviously, your current health status must be taken into account when planning exercise. Existing health problems will affect selection of type, duration, and frequency of exercise. Such problems will also place limits on how much improvement can be expected and at what rate. People with any current or potential health problem must be extremely careful in the beginning not to overstress their bodies. If you have some kind of cardiovascular problem, for example, especially close supervision of the program by a physician is essential. Frequent physical examinations are necessary to be sure that the exercise program is having a beneficial rather than a harmful effect.

In Chapter 3, there is a summary of medical considerations to take into account before you start an exercise program. If you have been very sedentary, a knowledgeable physician's observations and opinions are absolutely necessary. Even when cleared by the doctor, activity may be restricted to such exercises as walking, swimming, or bicycling. These activities are mild enough to be no danger to the cardiovascular system in most cases and will not predispose the body to major orthopedic problems.

Common sense will tell you, too, that when you have an illness such as a cold, minor infection, or injury, it is best to take a few days off. When you resume exercise after a temporary halt (for whatever reason), you should start at a lower work load and work your way up again.

BODY TYPE

People come in all shapes and sizes. Take a look around you. Some are fat, others thin, and some very muscular. Then there are all those people in between. Some are thin on top and heavy on the bottom or vice versa. The variations are endless.

To a certain extent, body type is permanent. You were born with a certain bone structure and build determined by your genes and chromosomes, and no amount of training or sport is going to alter it significantly.[2] Other factors, such as muscle composition and length of intestine, are inherited and unalterable. But if many of the current programs in physical education and recreation are an indication, people still take little account of the suitability of the human frame for particular exercises. There can be no joy for the lightly built person who is forced to participate in rugged contact sports. And there is nothing but frustration for the person who aspires to be a high jumper but is too heavy in the bone to win the fight against gravity.

Planning an exercise program without knowing your body type is sure to lead to problems. In many cases, matching exercise to body type can save time and money (for unused equipment, club memberships, lessons, etc.).

Scientists have attempted to classify the many varieties of human physique. Around 1940, a scientific basis for body typing—called "somatotyping"—was developed. Somatotyping is a method of classifying the body into three basic types (fat, muscular, and thin) by estimating the dominance of fat, bone, or muscle. According to Dr. W. H. Sheldon, a person is either an endomorph (round, soft body with little muscle development and small bones), a mesomorph (muscular and big-boned and noted for hardness and ruggedness), or an ectomorph (thin-muscled and boned, with a fragile and delicate body).[3] Of course, there are many variations and gradations of these three physical types. In fact, most people fall somewhere between the three extremes.

What has all this to do with your personal fitness program? Somatotyping is important because knowing your body type enables you to match your exercise routine to your body frame. For example, if you are a thin, small person (ectomorph), you are less buoyant than other types and probably more sensitive to temperature change; it is unlikely you will get the most out of—or even enjoy—a swimming program. Similarly, if you are on the heavy (endomorphic) side of the scale, you probably won't enjoy jogging long distances.

Research has shown that certain types of physique are

attracted to certain sports and exercise routines. Dr. Thomas K. Cureton, Ph.D., in his book *Physical Fitness Appraisal and Guidance,* points out that the active, wiry, relatively thin types (above average in ectomorphy) usually do best on endurance-type training such as long-distance running.[4] That's the person who can run five or ten or even twenty miles without feeling ill effects.

For people high in endomorphy, Dr. Cureton recommends low-powered activities such as bowling, sailing, bicycling, camping, swimming, tennis, badminton, shuffleboard, fishing, and skating. Both ectomorph and endomorph types should be encouraged to keep up their strength and cardiovascular condition, he adds.

Although mesomorphs as a rule have a relatively high physical fitness status, they tend to "drift" into an endomorph-type state. Dr. Cureton explains: "Such types get excessively fat very easily unless they can lead an active life with careful attention to diet." [5] They should try to cultivate avocations like gardening, sports, hiking, and camping, or a program of jogging mixed with continuous, rhythmical calisthenic-type exercises.

It all boils down to the fact that you can't do more than your body type—or somatotype—will allow. If you choose a workout routine that does not fit your body type, you can get away with it for a while, but sooner or later you'll simply give up (see Figure 9).

To put all this information to work for you, get yourself somatotyped. Many physical educators, fitness experts, and even YMCA physical directors are qualified to give you an accurate typing, but someone in your family can provide a rough estimate.

FIGURE 9 / BODY TYPE AND ACTIVITY PARTICIPATION

	PHYSICAL QUALITIES THAT ARE TYPICAL OF CERTAIN BODY TYPES					ACTIVITIES IN WHICH YOU CAN EXPECT TO EXPERIENCE MOST SUCCESS													
	Strength	Endurance	Power	Agility	Body Support	Archery	Badminton	Basketball	Bowling	Cycling	Golf	Handball	Hiking	Jogging	Skiing	Swimming	Tennis	Running	Wt. Training
Endomorphy																			
Meso-Endomorphy																			
Mesomorphy																			
Meso-Ectomorphy																			
Ectomorphy																			

"Body Type," in C. T. Kuntzleman (ed.), *The Physical Fitness Encyclopedia.* Emmaus, PA: Rodale Books, 1970, p. 58.

AGE

Age has already been mentioned as a factor in determining the ideal intensity for your exercise. The target pulse rate was highest for young people and decreased as age increased.

Age enters into exercise planning in other ways, too. If you maintain a physically active life-style during your developmental and middle years, you'll find that you probably can exercise vigorously even at a relatively old age.

It would be hard to disagree with Dr. Paul Dudley White, M.D.: "I'm sure that our health in middle age is very dependent upon what we do in our twenties. And I'm equally sure that the health at sixty, seventy, and eighty is very dependent on what we do in middle age." [6]

But what about people who have been inactive? What if you choose to become active after years of sedentary existence? Can you expect to benefit from, or even tolerate, vigorous exercise? In most cases, yes.

The period of maximum physical development is between the ages of twenty-five and thirty. After this, there is a slow decline in maximum strength, decreasing suddenly after fifty (but even at age sixty the loss does not usually exceed 20 percent of the maximum). Decline in speed of movement and reaction time show a similar pattern. Maximum heart rate, cardiac output (stroke volume times heart rate), and oxygen consumption also show a decline with age, with cardiac output at rest generally showing a decline of 1 percent after maturity.

These factors combined make for slower improvement and a lower rate of recovery from stress than what was experienced at an earlier age. Also, deconditioning (when inactive) takes place more rapidly and reconditioning progresses more slowly. Consequently, the overload, intensity, duration, and type of activity must be adapted accordingly. For older persons, strength, speed, and agility take on relatively less importance than flexibility, local muscle endurance, body weight, relaxation, and circulo-respiratory endurance. This should be reflected in the program. There is no current evidence that vigorous exercise will injure a healthy person, regardless of age. Proceed cautiously, realistically—and enthusiastically.

If you find that at the end of exercise you are extremely fatigued, then cut back the next day. If as you are exercising you find it difficult to hold a conversation with someone next to you, cut back. If at any time you are dizzy, suffer chest pains, exceptional fatigue, or pain—stop. If you find you are staggering, have mental confusion, lose facial color or have deep breathing or nausea, again cut back. Some of these should also be evaluated by a doctor.

Just remember: The older you are the longer it may take you to get into shape. You should spend more time on warm-up, and you should definitely listen to your body. But don't let anyone tell you you should get out of running and into the rocker. It just isn't so. Exercise is healthful and beneficial to the older citizen.[7]

SEX

It's ironic that popular culture prizes a shapely female figure and yet perpetuates the myth that exercise is unfeminine when exercise would, in fact, help women to maintain an attractive figure. It is an absurd situation. In reality, the entire spectrum of sports and exercise is open to both males and females. Specific fitness objectives are generally the same; all of the five components of fitness are to be developed and maintained in both men and women.

It has been reported that, on the average, women have a slightly lower fitness level than men in all the major components except flexibility. Research clearly points out, however, that the lower fitness level of females is probably due to cultural patterns (not encouraging women to exercise) rather than biological factors.[8] Dr. Jack Wilmore, Ph.D., observes that there is little difference in the strength, endurance, and body composition of male and female *athletes*. These women, of course, unlike most in modern America, *do* exercise regularly. For the general population, says Dr. Wilmore, the biggest difference between male and female fitness is in the strength of the upper body:

> Strength of the lower extremities, when related to body weight and lean body weight, is similar between the sexes, although the male maintains a distinct superiority in upper body strength. Weight lifting, formerly condemned as a mode of training for women because of its supposed masculinizing effects, is now recognized as extremely valuable and necessary in developing the strength component, which is usually the weak link in the physiological profile of the female athlete.[9]

Looking at highly trained distance runners, Dr. Wilmore finds that endurance fitness is comparable in males and females, provided that differences in lean body weight are taken into account. Body composition is also similar; the female is below the male in weight, but the ratio of fat to overall weight is similar to the male. Dr. Wilmore concludes: "Because of these similarities, and because their needs are essentially the same, there is little reason to advocate different training or conditioning programs on the basis of sex." [10]

Consumer Guide® deplores the prevalent tendency of American cultural patterns to overprotect women and discourage them from physical activity after puberty. The fitness needs of women are much the same as those of men: consequently, the guidelines set forth in this volume apply to both men and women.

IT'S IN YOUR HANDS

By now you've surely seen that selecting the exercise program that is just right for you is by no means simple. You have many things to think about; you have to meet the various needs of your one-of-a-kind body and you have to find a pleasing way to do it. Actually these goals are not so separate; once you get started and begin to develop your potential for fitness, the activity should prove to be satisfying as well as beneficial. Our aim is simply to provide you with information and guidelines to make your introduction to regular exercise as painless as possible and free of false starts and setbacks.

6

HOW EXERCISE
HELPS YOUR HEART

CORONARY HEART DISEASE IS AMERICA'S BIGGEST KILLER, claiming the lives of over 700,000 people annually. The disease causes 30 percent of all deaths of men forty to fifty-nine. It's been estimated that twelve million Americans are currently being treated for coronary heart disease while another twelve million are afflicted and are not even aware of it. This high rate of coronary disease is largely responsible for the relatively poor life expectancy rate of U.S. males (eighteenth among the countries of the world).

Lack of exercise is one of the twelve heart disease risk factors listed by the American Heart Association. The other eleven are heredity, sex, race, age, smoking, stress, hypertension, lipid (fats and similar substances) abnormalities, diet, electrocardiographic abnormalities, and diabetes mellitus.[1] The growing interest in exercise as a protective factor in heart disease is the result of the recognition that exercise can do more than minimize the lack-of-exercise factor itself: it can also affect several other risk factors associated with coronary heart disease. In several studies, for example, it has been shown that exercise may reduce blood pressure, blood fats, and possibly psychic stress and strains.

WHAT IS CORONARY HEART DISEASE?

The circulatory system consists of the heart, arteries, veins, and capillaries. It is the function of this system to circulate blood to all parts of the body. The blood, in turn, furnishes the tissues with oxygen and food materials and removes waste products.

The heart—the pump that forces blood through the arteries and veins—is composed of muscle tissue, called the myocardium. As with all body muscles, the heart tissue requires a continuous blood supply. This supply does not consist of the blood coursing through the heart chambers but is delivered through a special set of arteries, the coronary arteries, which surround and attach to the myocardium.

For some reason a condition called atherosclerosis develops in many people. Yellowish and whitish spots, called "atheromas," start to accumulate on the inner walls of the arteries. These consist of deposits of fatty substances (cholesterol). At the outset they are very small, little more than tiny marks on the lining of the vessels. Eventually, however, with greater accumulation, they begin to protrude into the inner surfaces of the blood vessels. Over a period of years, the atheromas enlarge substantially until they interfere with the free flow of blood.

Atheromas may occur in arteries anywhere in the body. When they are located in the coronary arteries and the blood supply to a particular region of the myocardium is blocked, the muscle in that region dies. This death of heart tissue, called a myocardial infarction, is commonly known as a heart attack. In some cases, the immediate cause of the attack is a blood clot, or thrombus, which blocks an artery already narrowed by atherosclerosis. This kind of heart attack is called a coronary thrombosis.

A pain or ache may persist after the initial blockage, for

the fibers of the heart that are not receiving oxygenated blood stop contracting and become swollen. These tissues die, and the pain subsides. The specific part of the heart that receives no oxygen has suffered an injury and requires time to heal. The rest of the heart (unless the heart attack is so severe it has caused death) continues to struggle along in a limited capacity.

Heart disease is a complicated ailment. Many factors are interrelated (obesity, diet, activity, blood fats, etc.), and it is important to remember that in isolating exercise we are looking at just one limited aspect of treatment of this disease. Within this book, the modest intent is to explore the potential role of exercise in helping to "manage" heart disease.

THE EVIDENCE OF POPULATION STUDIES

Numerous studies have been conducted comparing active and inactive populations with respect to coronary heart disease. When these studies are examined, it becomes apparent that people who maintain a relatively high level of occupational and recreational activity have a much lower incidence of heart attacks than those who do not. Moreover, the more active people seem to have a better chance of recovering from a heart attack.

Researchers in the United States have discovered that workers who perform a significant amount of physical labor as part of their work run less risk of coronary disease.

An early study by Dr. O. F. Hedley, M.D., compiled data on 5,116 deaths due to coronary occlusion in Philadelphia from 1933 through 1937. In comparing the coronary death rates of various occupational groups, it was seen that workers had a lower rate than did professional men, business managers, and clerks. The rates per 100,000 were 154 for professional men; 140 for business managers; 128 for clerks; and 107 for workers.[3]

In 1962, Dr. Henry L. Taylor, Ph.D., of the University of Minnesota investigated the relationship of physical activity to coronary heart disease among men aged forty through sixty-four in the railroad industry. This industry was selected because most railroad employees who are forty years of age or older have accumulated seniority in their jobs and remain railroad employees until retirement or death. Furthermore, changes in job classification within the industry are infrequent, and records of the Railroad Retirement Board are reasonably complete and accurate. The jobs the men performed, their physical activity classification, and total number of man-years were as follows: clerks, sedentary, 85,112; switchmen, moderately active, 61,630; section men, heavily active, 44,867. The total age-adjusted heart disease death rates per 1,000 were 5.7 for clerks, 3.9 for switchmen, and 2.8 for section men.[4]

In the Framingham, Massachusetts, study a U.S. Public Health Service team classified men according to habitual physical activity and their subsequent incidence of coronary heart disease over a period of ten years. During this period of ten years, 207 men developed some form of a coronary attack. Those classified most sedentary in each age group had a coronary incidence almost twice that of those who were at least moderately active.[5]

In 1951, a large group of San Francisco longshoremen were given screening examinations that included assessment of characteristics related to degenerative cardiovascular disease. Sixteen years later, a follow-up was conducted on 3,263 of these men. A total of 888 deaths had occurred; 291 of these fatalities, or 33 percent, were from coronary heart disease. Men with physically less active jobs died of coronaries one-third more frequently than those in more physically demanding cargo-handling positions. When comparisons of coronary deaths were made by age, the favorable effect associated with job activity was greatest at the youngest and decreased steadily to disappearance at the oldest age. Other important risk factors found to be related to coronary fatalities were cigarette smoking and high systolic blood pressure.[6]

In Westchester County, New York, postmortem studies (conducted over a period of ten years) revealed that the age at death of men who had engaged in sedentary occupations was generally lower than those whose occupations involved a good bit of physical activity. In this study, bank executives, clerks, accountants, and taxi drivers were noted as sedentary; grocery clerks and letter carriers were regarded as moderately active; and road construction workers, plumbers, and steamfitters were considered strenuously active. The percentages of sudden deaths from heart attacks under age fifty-five according to physical activity classification were 44 percent for the sedentary occupations, 31 percent for the moderate, and 24 percent for strenuous.[7]

A more recent study by Doctors R. S. Paffenbarger, Jr., M.D., and W. E. Hale, M.D.,[8] compared men who did heavy, moderate, and light longshoreman's work. The doctors concluded that those workers classified as "heavy workers" had significantly lower death rates from coronary heart disease. The investigators also stated that the difference between the groups persisted when five other risk factors were taken into account—cigarette smoking, systolic blood pressure, body weight, diagnosed heart disease, and glucose metabolism.

THE 1973 MORRIS STUDY (REGARDING RECREATIONAL HABITS)

In 1973, Dr. J. N. Morris and his associates of the Medical Research Council Social Medicine Unit, London School of Hygiene and Tropical Medicine, reported on an extensive survey of the effects of recreational exercise on the heart. Instead of comparing the incidence of heart disease among people in physically active and inactive occupations, the researchers built their survey around the relative amount of leisure-time exercise, noting that "work in advanced societies is increasingly light and sedentary, so any future contribution to public health can only come from exercise taken in leisure time." [9]

Aware, too, of certain criticisms of previous studies, the British team sent their questionnaire to 16,882 middle-aged men in government executive-grade positions, all of them engaged in sedentary or physically very light work. The men were requested to give an account of their physical activity for each five minutes of two days, a Friday (normally working) and Saturday (free), the record being completed on the following Monday morning and then returned directly to the research team. The selected days were unannounced so the behavior would not be influenced and the "recall" method was preferred to the "diary" for the same reason.

Next, the activities of the men were analyzed. "Vigorous" activities were defined as those likely to reach peaks of energy output corresponding to heavy industrial work, thus producing a training effect on the cardiovascular system. These included active recreation such as swimming, keep-fit exercises, heavy work (digging), and "getting around quickly"—running, jogging, and walking. That phase of the study was concluded in 1970.

By 1972, about 232 of the men surveyed had suffered a first clinical attack of coronary disease. The researchers then matched each of these heart disease patients with two "controls" not so affected. To eliminate biases as a result of personal, social, and environmental factors, the controls were men of the same age within one year, the same job classification, the same geographical region, similar family composition, and comparable worldly goods, smoking habits, and diet patterns.

"During the two sample days," Dr. Morris explains,

"eleven percent of the men who developed coronary disease, compared with twenty-six percent of the controls, reported vigorous activity. In men recording vigorous exercise the relative risk of developing coronary disease was about a third that in comparable men who did not, and in men reporting much of it still less. Vigorous exercise apparently protected against rapid fatal heart attacks and other first clinical attacks of coronary disease alike, throughout middle age." [10]

LIMITATIONS OF POPULATION SURVEYS

Population studies are quite limited, of course. Although they do show that more active populations suffer less often and less severely from coronary heart disease, it is possible that individuals who are more active may also be more aware of good general health practices.

Another problem associated with these studies stems from the many definitions of "physical activity." For some people, physical activity means running several miles; for others it's a round of golf once a week. Consequently, almost none of the exercise measured in the "active versus inactive" comparisons was endurance-type exercise. Extensive as they are, the population studies are not the whole story.

HOW EXERCISE CONDITIONS THE CIRCULATORY SYSTEM

The population studies provide ample indication that exercise is related in some way to lower risk of heart disease. But how? What are the mechanisms by which habitual physical activity may reduce the occurrence or severity of coronary heart disease? Dr. Samuel Fox,[11] past president of the American Cardiology Society, suggests a few of the more important factors.

CORONARY COLLATERAL VASCULATION (OPENING UP OF NEW BLOOD VESSELS TO HEART TISSUE)

Dr. Fox suggests that physical exercise may be a factor in the development of passages carrying oxygenated blood around coronary obstructions. It has long been speculated that when a coronary artery supplying blood to a portion of the heart muscle is blocked, changes may occur in the coronary network, enabling blood from other arteries to reach the affected portion of the myocardium. Tiny new arteries bypass the blocked or narrowed artery. Dr. Fox points out that experiments with animals indicate that exercise is a significant factor in the appearance of this "collateral circulation." For example, dogs kept inactive either fail to develop collateral circulation or develop less of it than do dogs that are exercised daily.[12]

The studies conducted on humans have not been as conclusive and the evidence is fragmentary, but we do know that some middle-aged persons with coronary obstructions develop collaterals. They form occasionally with or without exercise. This phenomenon of new blood vessels opening to supply damaged heart tissue is of the greatest interest to scientists. Although it's not likely that an adequate flow can develop in extensive ("three-vessel") coronary obstructions, it may be that, where just one vessel is involved, collaterals can expand from relatively uninvolved arteries nearby.[13]

MYOCARDIAL (HEART MUSCLE) EFFICIENCY

One of the most apparent benefits of regular exercise is improved myocardial efficiency—greater work performed at a lesser cost. As you become physically trained, your heart supplies the body's needs with a decreasing number of beats per minute—at rest and at every level of physical activity. More blood is pumped per stroke. The increase in stroke volume is thought to require, for a given work load, a lesser amount of myocardial oxygen. In addition, the increased cardiac output (amount of blood pumped each minute) is distributed more efficiently. This improved power function of the myocardium (a stronger pump with more horsepower) is one of the most important aspects of training. It enables your heart to respond to sudden demand more efficiently and more safely; the trained heart can pump more blood with each beat than the untrained heart.

IMPROVED MAXIMUM OXYGEN UPTAKE

"Maximum oxygen uptake" refers to the body's ability to pick up, transport, and utilize oxygen. Improvement in this area is another adaptive mechanism by which physical training can improve the working of your heart. The maximum oxygen uptake is a measure of the amount of oxygen used by the body during exhausting exercise—such as an all-out run. It reflects both the ability of the ventricles to put out an increased stroke volume and the distribution of the increased cardiac output. This measurement corresponds to the upper limit of aerobic work capacity. Many studies have shown that it can be improved through endurance-type training such as walking, jogging, swimming, or cycling.

BALANCED MYOCARDIAL HORMONE PRODUCTION

According to Dr. Fox,[14] during periods of emotional stress and other kinds of excitement the adrenal glands are stimulated to release selected hormones. These hormones increase the need of the heart muscle for oxygen. The normal heart responds with an increase in heartbeat and blood flow.

The trained myocardium is more efficient in response to this increased oxygen need and there is less oxygen wastage, primarily resulting from a decrease in myocardial hormones.

In the untrained heart, or in the presence of coronary artery disease, this protective mechanism may fail, resulting in an under-supply of oxygen ("hypoxia"). This, in turn, causes depletion of cardiac magnesium and potassium and increase in sodium content. The imbalance may aggravate the hypoxia and create a vicious cycle. With these conditions, cardiac conduction and contractability are distorted with the consequent likelihood of abnormal heartbeat, inadequate blood supply, or congestive heart failure.

CHOLESTEROL AND OTHER SERUM LIPIDS

Chemically, cholesterol is an organic substance belonging to a group of crystalline or solid alcohols known as sterols. It serves as a structural component of nerve tissue and plays a role in the formation of vitamin D_3 and the body steroids. Thus, this substance is essential to the individual well-being; yet it can also be a cause of heart disease. High cholesterol levels have been associated with coronary heart disease.

The relationship between physical activity and serum lipid levels, especially serum cholesterol, has not been established. Although numerous studies have indicated that exercise may have a beneficial effect on reducing cholesterol, some others have produced conflicting results.

Dr. Thomas K. Cureton, Ph.D., believes that some of the differences obtained in conflicting studies is due to the type of exercise program administered. He concluded that exercise reduces cholesterol in the blood serum when the work is long enough, hard enough, and of a cardiovascular endurance type. Easy programs are relatively ineffective—bowling, golf, leisurely walking, casual swimming, and games played intermittently, such as softball and volleyball.

Some cholesterol reductions occur when one participates in more strenuous activities such as interval-style walk/jog, and games like tennis, handball, and squash. The programs found best for cholesterol reduction were continuous—running, swimming, skating, skiing, cycling, hiking, and competitive games in which weight is lost and a negative caloric balance occurs.[15] Dr. Cureton's findings support the crucial importance of cardiovascular exercise.

Another possibility is that exercise is effective in reducing cholesterol levels over the long range, with little short-term effect. Dr. Jean Mayer, Ph.D., of Harvard thinks this is so. He and Dr. Daniella Gsell studied the residents of Blattendorf, a village in the Swiss Alps, several miles from the nearest cart path. "All distances have to be walked," Dr. Mayer reports. "The people carry hay, wood, milk, and building materials on their backs. Men frequently carry loads of fifty or sixty pounds up and down the mountain paths." These mountain dwellers eat precisely the kind of diet—high in animal fats and dairy products—associated with high cholesterol levels. Yet their cholesterol levels are very low. Dr. Mayer concluded that despite the negative evidence, physical activity over a period of years may prove to be a factor in lowering cholesterol levels.[16]

ARTERIAL BLOOD PRESSURE

Dr. John L. Boyer, M.D., is one cardiologist who has been most outspoken in the belief that exercise can play a role in reducing high blood pressure. The study he and Dr. Fred Kasch, Ph.D., did several years ago illustrates the point. Doctors Boyer and Kasch put twenty-three middle-aged men with high blood pressure and twenty-two with normal blood pressure on a six-month exercise training program. The routine consisted of fifteen to twenty minutes of warm-up exercise, followed by walking/jogging. All of these men had been inactive before the program, and no attempt was made to alter their diet. At the end of six months there were significant reductions in the blood pressures of the hypertensive men. There were no changes reported for the normal group.[17]

The evidence is far from conclusive, and other observers are skeptical about improving blood pressure through cardiovascular exercise, but contemporary thinking and research at least suggest a possibility that deserves attention.

Dr. Kenneth Cooper, M.D.,[18] and his associates conducted an interesting study on risk factors and fitness levels. Approximately 3,000 men with an average age of 44.6 years were evaluated. The evaluation included a blood and lipid profile, blood pressure, body fat, treadmill time, and some selected pulmonary functions. According to the authors: "A consistent inverse relationship among physical fitness categories and resting heart rate, body weight, percent body fat, serum levels of cholesterol and triglycerides, glucose, and systolic blood pressure was observed." In plain English, as the fitness level of the subjects went up, the risk factors (cholesterol, triglycerides, blood pressure, glucose, uric acid, and percent fat) went down.

THE VERDICT: EXERCISE AND YOUR HEART

On the whole, it is clear that cardiovascular efficiency is closely related to physical fitness and regular exercise. Exercise is not the only factor of importance, of course. We would not even go as far as to claim that it is most important. Clearly, you can't build a strong heart with exercise alone, but then again, you probably can't have a strong heart without exercising it regularly.

7

EXERCISE AND
WEIGHT CONTROL

As our society becomes more mechanized, weight control will become more and more difficult. We give much lip service to physical activity, then do everything possible to program it out of our lives. We ride when we could walk, use elevators or escalators instead of stairs, and keep looking for even easier ways to perform daily tasks.

THE MODERN ROAD TO OVERWEIGHT

Every cut in physical activity is significant. If a secretary switches from a manual typewriter to an electric typewriter, she burns just a few calories less per hour. But the change is enough that in one year's time the typist will gain six pounds! Every extension phone in a home saves seventy miles of walking; for the average person, this means a two-pound weight increase each year. Compare, too, the amount of energy (calories) spent using old-fashioned tools and devices with the energy expended using today's push-button models.

When was the last time you saw anyone outdoors at a clothesline beating the dust out of a rug? Electric vacuum cleaners do the job now; outdoor models even suck up leaves. You don't have to work up a sweat raking and bundling leaves; if you don't have an outdoor vacuum cleaner, you probably have a power mower with an attachment to take care of the leaves. You may not even have to stand up to guide it; if your power mower is a midget tractor model, you just sit on it and steer it smoothly across the lawn. It's great for your grass—but not for your health.

Thanks to your refrigerator or freezer, you don't have to expend energy chopping ice blocks as in the days of the wooden ice boxes. If you want to paint the outside of your house, you certainly don't need to move a paint brush back and forth; just spray the surface with an electric power sprayer.

Yes, modern society has made it extremely easy to gain weight and very difficult to take it off.

It's not hard to find weight-control "experts" who are doubtful of the effectiveness of exercise as a method of weight-reduction. Two misconceptions persist—first, that exercise requires relatively little caloric expenditure and is, therefore, ineffective in weight control; and second, that exercise increases the appetite and is self-defeating as a weight-control method.

CALORIE-SPENDING THROUGH EXERCISE

The body maintains a fine balance between the number of calories eaten and the number burned off through physical activity. For example, if a person takes in 2,400 calories of food and burns off 2,400 calories during sleeping, eating, working, walking, etc., he will maintain his body weight. But if he eats 2,400 calories per day and burns off only 2,300, he will have 100 calories left over. Those excess calories will then be stored as fat in the fat cells in the body until they are needed.

Skeptics point out that it takes a great deal of exercise to burn off the caloric equivalent of one pound of fat—for example, thirty-six miles of walking, seven hours of splitting wood, eleven hours of playing volleyball, or six hours of playing handball.

The flaw in this reasoning is that these equations completely ignore the *cumulative effect of exercise*. We have no trouble recognizing the cumulative nature of weight gain. Physiologists tell us that approximately 3,500 calories equal one pound of fat. It doesn't matter what type of food is eaten—calories are calories, and they *do* count. Therefore, an extra 100 calories a day will add up to one pound in thirty-five days. By the end of the year, approximately ten pounds will have been gained.

This sort of slow gain has been called "creeping obesity." Usually weight gain is noticed over a period of months or years, not overnight. One year you buy a 36-inch belt; you need a 38-inch one the next year.

Now turn this process around. What about "creeping fat loss"? It may indeed take six hours of handball to burn up one pound of fat, but it need not be a single six-hour period. One half-hour of handball every day for twelve days would also burn one pound of fat; playing handball at that rate would burn up thirty to thirty-six pounds of fat in a single year.

There is another interesting way to look at this misconception regarding the number of calories used up in exercise. It is recognized that people who engage in intense physical activity need extra caloric intake to "fuel" the activity. For example, the "caloric requirements" tables of the U.S. National Research Council recommend 2,400 calories daily for "sedentary" men and 4,500 calories for "very active" men. The NRC advises laborers, soldiers, and athletes that they may require up to (and occasionally more than) 6,000 calories a day.[1] If engaging in intense activity means you must double your usual calorie intake, then it must follow, by reverse logic, that such exertion does use calories to a significant degree.

EXERCISE AND APPETITE

The second misconception regarding exercise is that an increase in physical activity is self-defeating in weight control because it increases appetite. Exercise does indeed increase the appetite of normally active people, but this is the body's protective mechanism. Without it, obviously the body of a person who plays handball for half an hour a day, thereby expending the caloric equivalent of thirty to thirty-six pounds a year, would burn away to nothing over a period of three or four years. The increase in hunger makes it possible to exercise without undermining well-being.

But the principle does *not* work in reverse. Decreasing activity below a moderate level will not decrease the appetite. In fact, appetite has been seen to increase with inactivity. Thus, under-exercising rather than overeating may be the more important cause of overweight.

Observations of both laboratory animals and human beings support the belief that under-exercising causes weight gains. In the Nutrition Department of Harvard University, Dr. Jean Mayer, Ph.D., and his colleagues studied the relationship between food intake, exercise, and weight in white mice. The research team accustomed a large group of mice to running on a motor-driven treadmill. The mice were then separated into small groups, and each group was exercised for a fixed period of time each day, ranging from one to ten hours daily. The doctors measured food intake and recorded weight changes for each group of mice, and then compared the results with similar data for a control group of mice which had not been exercised.

The research team found that the sedentary control group of mice ate *more* than the moderately active group (those which exercised for one or two hours daily) and slowly accumulated weight. The mice that exercised the most consumed more food than the moderately active groups, but their weight stabilized at a lower level than that of both the sedentary and moderately active mice. The moderately active mice ate less than the sedentary and very active mice. Their weight was less than that of the sedentary mice, but slightly more than the very active mice.[2]

Some years ago, a comparable study was made of an industrial population in Calcutta. At one end of the scale were the supervisors and clerks, extremely sedentary individuals who sat throughout their work hours. In the middle were the mechanics, drivers, weavers, and others whose work called for an average amount of physical exertion. At the other end of the scale were the ashmen, coalmen, blacksmiths, cutters and carriers—extremely active people who carried heavy loads (roughly equal to their body weight) for eight to nine hours daily. The results of the study were similar to those in the work with mice. The sedentary merchants and clerks ate only a little more than the moderately active people but weighed considerably more. And although the very active blacksmiths, carriers, ashmen, and others ate as much as the sedentary merchants did, on the average they weighed fourteen pounds less. The moderately active employees ate less than the sedentary and weighed less.[3]

Weight control depends on a proper balance between calorie consumption and physical activity. As we've seen, the level of activity of most modern life-styles is minimal, and it takes a deliberate decision of will for us to increase our physical activity through selected sports and exercise.

THE ROLE OF HUNGER

Hunger is perhaps one of the most misunderstood words in our vocabulary. Hunger refers to the craving for food that is usually associated with a number of unpleasant sensations. The person who has had no food for many hours will have stomach contractions, often called hunger pains. They produce a gnawing sensation that we have all experienced when we've skipped breakfast and lunchtime approaches. Most of us, however, have never known the severe pain of acute hunger suffered by millions of starving people around the world. Therefore, most of us do not understand true hunger.

The term *appetite* is often confused with hunger. Appetite refers to the desire for a specific type of food, such as strawberries, milk, cake, cookies, soda, etc. Appetite determines the kind of food a person eats.

Satiety is the opposite of both hunger and appetite. It means complete fulfillment—the absence of both hunger and appetite—even though food may be available.

All of these terms—hunger, appetite, and satiety—refer to complex sensations that determine eating habits.

The stomach does not control hunger. Even people who have had part or all of their stomach removed continue to experience hunger just as before. Hunger is a response to the fluctuating glucose level of the blood in the brain. Scientists call this phenomenon the "glucostatic regulation of food intake." [4] Although there are still missing links in the theory of this phenomenon, it has more scientific evidence to support it than does any other concept.

THE GLUCOSTATIC THEORY

Among the many important functions of the hypothalamus, a tiny area at the base of the brain, is the regulation of hunger. The hunger impulse is a reaction to either the presence or lack of glucose in the blood.

Simply stated, the "glucostatic theory" asserts that when the blood glucose concentration falls too low, the ventromedial hypothalamus (the part that signals satiety) reduces its inhibiting effects on the lateral hypothalamus (which controls the hunger sensation). Consequently, an impulse is sent from the lateral hypothalamus to the cerebral cortex of the brain and from the cortex to the stomach, where gastric contractions begin, thus causing the feeling of hunger.

What is *not* known is what determines either the size of the meal eaten or the sense of fullness after a meal. Speculation is that there are receptors of some type in the gastrointestinal tract that may trigger a nervous or hormonal mechanism that activates the hypothalamic satiety center. Factors that may trigger such a process include taste and smell, the number of fat deposits on the body, amino acid imbalance, glucose released by the liver, and glucagon (a protein that elevates the blood glucose levels).

Calories (found only in proteins, fats, and carbohydrates) are essential, therefore, to satisfy hunger for any period of time. Bulk has very little to do with satisfying hunger. The sense of fullness that many people experience when they eat low- or noncaloric foods may be due to receptors in the gastro-intestinal tract, but the feeling of fullness does not last long. This prompts the old saying that certain foods don't "stick to your ribs."

This is a serious indictment of noncaloric food sources. People who use diet sodas, soups, crackers, cookies, etc., in an effort to reduce weight are just kidding themselves. They may lose weight in the initial stages of the diet, but their hunger will continue because of low glucose levels. As a result they will be continually hungry.

Scientific experiments illustrate this phenomenon. In one classic example rats were given a certain amount of food over a period of time. Activity and diet were maintained at a constant level, and the rats were able to hold a steady weight. The researchers then changed 10 percent of the diet to material that contained no calories—food very similar to that used by people who are dieting. It was found that when the new food contained 10 percent inert material, the rats ate approximately 10 percent more food. When the researchers raised the noncaloric portion to 20 percent, the animals ate 20 percent more food. This trend continued as the proportion of noncaloric food was increased. Finally, the animals literally ate themselves to death attempting to satisfy their appetite with low-calorie, high-bulk foods.[5]

The glucostatic theory explains why some foods satisfy hunger and others don't. But it is still not clear why some people crave more food than others and seem to be hungry all the time. Many theories, however, have been postulated in an effort to explain this.

THE APPESTAT THEORY

Scientists and lay people refer to the feeding and satiety center of the hypothalamus as the *appestat*. It has been suggested that this center of regulation may be "set" a little higher in some people than in others. A person whose appestat has a higher setting is usually one who has greater difficulty in controlling weight. Although experiencing both hunger and satiety, the person with a high setting needs a little more food (glucose, to which all proteins, carbohydrates, or fats are eventually converted) to satisfy the satiety center, or appestat. Exactly why the appestat is set higher is not clear, but many scientists feel that the concept of the appestat is one that fits into the human evolutionary scheme. The theory also provides perhaps one of the most logical explanations of why people gain weight.

In primitive cultures human beings had to be physically active to survive. A high appestat setting was an advantage; a person with a higher setting, for example, experienced greater hunger and pursued food much more avidly than a person with a lower setting. As a result, more food was obtained, eaten, and stored, so that his or her body had additional energy at hand and more body tissue. During periods when little or no food could be found, stored body fat and tissue provided sustenance until an animal was slain or some other food found. The person with the lower appestat setting had less stored energy and body tissue. It is important to note that the person physically active in the pursuit and preparation of food never became obese.

In modern Western society the situation is reversed. Vigorous physical activity is no longer required to obtain and prepare food, but we still have appestats. Nowadays, if you are a person with the higher appestat setting you are at a disadvantage. The evolutionary instinct to eat more food so that you will be able to survive in a period of crisis continues to operate, but today you are likely to be under-exercised. You don't burn up the excess calories, so you gain weight. And, unless you become marooned on a desert island, no nutritional crisis will occur in your lifetime. So the pounds will continue to add up.

You can, of course, restrict your caloric intake, but you will experience a continual hunger, a hunger that is constantly stimulated by food ads on TV, radio, billboards, and in magazines and newspapers. Your appestat will demand that the hunger be satisfied. Since hunger is satisfied by increasing caloric intake, unless you are extremely strong-willed, practically any diet is doomed to failure.

THE PSYCHOLOGICAL THEORY

The psychological theory of weight gain is also widely accepted by professional and lay people in this field. Its advocates maintain that obesity and overweight are by-products of psychological problems.

A researcher can cause a rat to overeat by punishing it if it does not. This kind of conditioning occurs in human beings, too. Many children eat and overeat in an effort to win their parents' approval, or, in some cases, to avoid actual punishment. Some well-meaning parents still believe that "a fat child is a healthy child" and insist that their children overeat. Also, some parents and other adults give children cookies or candy as a reward for good behavior, or to distract them from crying after a fall.

The first exposure to overeating often occurs very early in life. Dr. Hilde Bruch, M.D., Professor of Psychiatry at Baylor College of Medicine, states that a baby's tears are often misinterpreted as hunger. Unfortunately, many adults thrust a bottle in the mouth of a crying infant instead of considering whether the need may be for cuddling, comfort, a diaper change, or a change of scene. Therefore, it's only natural that the child learns to link emotional and physical needs with eating.[6] If food is used to placate needs other than hunger, a child may be "conditioned" to want food even when not hungry.

Another aspect of the psychological theory focuses on the role of tension and frustration in overeating. Usually stress situations (death of a parent, loss of a job, etc.) cause you to eat nervously, if you were so conditioned in childhood, and also to refrain from physical activity. In fact, you may want to sleep more, or you may become depressed and just want to sit.

The most interesting aspect of the psychological theory is the observation that obese/overweight people tend to become less active, thereby compounding the problem. Dr. Albert Stunkard, M.D., has observed that situations that cause overeating also lead to decreased physical activity, and that a person who experiences periods of intense depression may also undergo a significant change in carbohydrate metabolism.[7]

Obesity/overweight contributes to inactivity, and inactivity begets weight gain; it is indeed a "vicious circle." Dr. M. F. Graham, M. D., of Dallas, Texas, has illustrated that cycle in a diagram (Figure 10).

The Graham diagram shows the usual progression: stress, anxiety, and tension lead to compulsive eating, which shows up as fat (obesity/overweight), which leads to physical inactivity, and therefore greater stress, anxiety, and tension. Physical activity is the simplest means of breaking the vicious cycle outlined by Dr. Graham. Physical activity is the way to control body weight.

FIGURE 10 / THE OVEREATING CYCLE

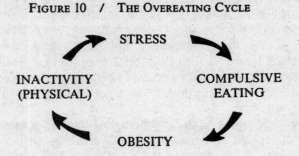

M. F. Graham, *Prescription For Life*. New York: David McKay, 1966, p. 43.

Both the appestat and psychological theories are valid. In fact, in many instances obesity and overweight result from a combination of causes. What you must remember is that *physical activity is the most reliable way to control weight.*

EXERCISE WORKS BEST

Many times when people lose weight through dieting they complain that they still look flabby. And they do. That is because they lose weight—fat *and* lean body tissue. As you know, fat is fat, but lean body tissue is the bone/muscle tissue of your body. The lean body tissue gives you your shape—and that you don't want to lose. Exercise is superior to dieting because it results not only in weight loss, but also in fat loss, and there is no loss in lean body tissue.

Doctors Bill Zuti, Ph.D., and Lawrence Golding, Ph.D., conducted a study that illustrates this point nicely. The research team set out to compare the effect of several different methods of weight reduction on body weight, body composition, and selected blood measurements. The twenty-five women participating in the study were all between the ages of twenty-five and forty and were twenty to forty pounds overweight. Three groups were formed: (1) eight women were on a diet, reducing their caloric intake by 500 calories per day, but holding their physical activity constant; (2) nine continued to eat as usual, but increased physical activity to burn off 500 extra calories a day; and (3) eight reduced caloric intake by 250 calories a day and increased physical activity to burn off 250 calories per day. Before and after the sixteen-week period, the subjects were tested for body weight, body density, skin-fold and girth measurements, and selected blood lipids (fats).

The results indicated that there was no significant difference between the groups in the amount of weight loss. The average individual weight loss in all three groups was 11.4 pounds. Thus, the study indicated that all of the methods were extremely effective in controlling weight. However, the significant finding of the study was that there was a difference between the groups with regard to body composition. Those in the exercise group and in the combination exercise/diet group had undergone significant changes in body density. The dieting group lost both body fat and muscle tissue; the exercise group lost more body fat and no muscle tissue.

In the study by Golding and Zuti, the members of the exercise group also had more stamina than the others; their circulatory systems were much better able to withstand the rigors of exercise. The report concluded that the use of exercise in a weight-reduction program is far superior to dieting alone in its effect on body composition and physical fitness.[8]

When people lose weight by dieting they often remain flabby. But if you exercise while you diet or use exercise as the means of losing weight, your muscles will be much firmer. Therefore, you will look and feel better after losing weight through exercising than you will after just dieting.

8

AEROBICS AND OTHER CARDIOVASCULAR EXERCISE PROGRAMS

THANKS TO DR. KENNETH COOPER, M.D., AND HIS BOOK *Aerobics,*[1] practically every fitness book published since 1968 makes mention of aerobic exercise. It may be praised, condemned, or simply described, but it cannot be ignored.

The idea that a certain type of exercise can "condition" the heart and lungs was not new. A long list of highly respected physicians and physiologists had been writing and speaking about cardiovascular exercise for years. Among them were Robert T. McKenzie, A. V. Hill, A. B. Bock, D. B. Dill, E. C. Schneider, Paul Dudley White, Joseph Wolffe, Thomas K. Cureton, Bruno Balke, and Per-Olaf Åstrand. Four books emphasizing cardiovascular exercise—*Physical Fitness and Dynamic Health*[2] (1965), *The Healthy Life*[3] (1966), *Prescription For Life*[4] (1966), and *Jogging*[5] (1967)—had already met with some popular success.

It was Cooper's book, however, that caught the attention of the public and made "aerobics" a household word. Many explanations have been given for the success of this particular book. The timing was perfect, for one thing; the earlier work on cardiovascular exercise had set the stage. Dr.

Cooper presented the arguments in favor of cardiovascular exercise clearly and concisely, in terms that practically everyone could understand and accept. The fact that his research was carefully documented (unusual in fitness books) strengthened his arguments. Many readers especially appreciated his system of equating certain types of exercise, which made it easy to compare exercises. Whatever the reason, one thing is clear: Kenneth Cooper has done more to popularize cardiovascular exercise than any other person in the world.

This chapter will focus on programs that emphasize cardiovascular exercise exclusively—without reference to pulse rate. Later chapters will discuss other programs that refer to pulse-rated exercise and cardiovascular exercise with calisthenics. In still another chapter, we will consider some weight control programs with a cardiovascular emphasis.

DR. KENNETH COOPER'S AEROBIC EXERCISE PLANS

Dr. Kenneth Cooper has written four books on aerobic exercise—*Aerobics* [6] (1968), *The New Aerobics* [7] (1970), *Aerobics for Women* [8] (1972), and *The Aerobics Way* (1977). In the last two, he expanded the exercise options and adjusted the program for age and sex.

AEROBICS

According to Kenneth Cooper, aerobics means literally "with oxygen." Aerobic exercises "are the foundation exercises on which any exercise program should be built. These exercises demand oxygen without producing an intolerable oxygen debt, so that they can be continued for long periods. They activate the training effect and start producing all those wonderful changes in your body." [9] Your lungs will process more air with less effort, your heart will grow stronger and pump more blood with each beat, the number and size of the blood vessels carrying blood to the body tissues will be increased, tone of the blood vessels and muscles will be improved, and your total blood volume will increase.

Cooper admits that he didn't discover or create any new exercises. He wanted to determine which of many alternative activities are best for the heart. His approach was to measure the amount of oxygen used during various activities, performed at varying intensities (duration and rate of speed), and then convert the measurements into a point system. (Remember the linear relationship between heart rate and oxygen consumed described in Chapter 4?)

For example, in Cooper's program running or walking one mile in 14½ to 20 minutes costs approximately seven milliliters of oxygen per kilogram of body weight per minute and is given the equivalent of one point, whereas running the mile between 6½ and 8 minutes costs approximately thirty-five milliliters of oxygen per kilogram per minute and has a value of five points. Other activities that count five points are swimming 600 yards in less than 15 minutes; cycling five miles in less than 20 minutes; stationary running for a total of 12½ minutes; and handball playing for 35 minutes.

Cooper concluded that a minimum of thirty points each week is necessary to produce or maintain cardiovascular fitness. You can't earn all the points in one day. They must be divided into three or four sessions. (See Figure 11 for a sample of his point charts.)

These principles were basic to all three of Dr. Cooper's books. The primary difference among the books was that he became more cautious with each one, scaled down the importance of his fitness field test, and adjusted the program for age and sex. And he revamped his point system slightly.

FIGURE 11 / SAMPLE CONDITIONING CHART: RUNNING

WEEK	DISTANCE (MILES/ SESSION)	WALK/RUN	TIME GOAL (MINUTES/ SESSION)	FREQ/WK	POINTS/WK
1	1.0	Walk	13:30	5	10
2	1.0	Walk	13:00	5	10
3	1.0	Walk	12:45	5	10
4	1.0	W/R	11:45	5	15
5	1.0	W/R	11:00	5	15
6	1.0	W/R	10:30	5	15
7	1.0	Run	9:45	5	20
8	1.0	Run	9:30	5	20
9	1.0	Run	9:15	5	20
10	1.0 and	Run	9:00	3	21
	1.5	Run	16:00	2	
11	1.0 and	Run	8:45	3	21
	1.5	Run	15:00	2	
12	1.0 and	Run	8:30	3	24
	1.5	Run	14:00	2	
13	1.0 and	Run	8:15	3	24
	1.5	Run	13:30	2	
14	1.0 and	Run	7:55	3	27
	1.5	Run	13:00	2	
15	1.0 and	Run	7:45	2	30
	1.5 and	Run	12:30	2	
	2.0	Run	18:00	1	
16	1.5 and	Run	11:55	2	31
	2.0	Run	17:00	2	

Kenneth H. Cooper, *Aerobics,* NY: M. Evans, 1968, p. 2.

THE NEW AEROBICS

In *The New Aerobics,* Cooper made several adjustments as a result of findings in his own research and criticism from the medical community. He had been somewhat casual in *Aerobics* about recommending a physical check-up before a person began an exercise program. He also emphasized to the reader to take his twelve-minute fitness test (how far can you run/walk in that time) prior to embarking on his program. But in *The New Aerobics,* he became a bit more cautious and specific. He recommended a medical checkup and played down the self-testing. "The main objective of this examination [the doctor's] is to spot heart, lung, and blood vessel problems that could make exercise potentially dangerous. This is especially important for older persons who are more likely to be affected by such problems." [10] He was quite specific about the type of examination necessary, and he also provided guidelines for several age groups.

In *The New Aerobics,* fitness testing became optional. "You can put yourself in fine shape without ever taking any test at all," he states. "Just follow the conditioning charts. By the time you reach the thirty-point-per-week level, just take it for granted that you're in good condition." [11] Figure 11 is a sample of one of his many conditioning charts. By carefully following the time and distance suggestions week by week, you can work your way up to the recommended thirty-point level.

An important addition in *The New Aerobics* was the six-week starter program for beginners. Another was the list of over twenty specific physical conditions that preclude individuals from exercising. All of these were excellent changes.

Cooper also called attention in this second book to certain age restrictions, pointing out that aerobic exercise can slow down but not undo some of the deterioration associated with aging. The person between thirty and fifty years of age can engage in almost any activity, needing a doctor's specific approval only for the most strenuous (running, jogging, etc.). Cooper recommended that the fifty- to fifty-nine-year-olds start by using the walking program to condition the body before considering running, jogging, or a more demanding competitive sport such as basketball, handball, or squash. Here again, a doctor's approval was recommended before beginning the more arduous activities. The alternative for this age group was to choose the less strenuous exercises, such as walking, golf, cycling (particularly stationary cycling), and swimming.

Cooper cautioned the sixty-and-over group (except those who have exercised regularly for years and are in top shape) to avoid jogging, running, and vigorous competitive sports and recommended instead walking, swimming, and stationary cycling.[12]

AEROBICS FOR WOMEN

Aerobics for Women was a further development of *Aerobics* and *The New Aerobics*. In it Dr. Cooper and his wife Mildred applied the concepts presented in the first two books to women.

The authors make a distinction between male and female motivation in beginning to exercise. They accept the view that women, more often than men, exercise for cosmetic reasons—to get into a certain dress size or improve their figure. Men, on the other hand, may exercise for cosmetic reasons, but their primary concern is usually coronary heart disease. Furthermore, the Coopers had observed that most American women disliked jogging (this attitude is apparently far less common today) and preferred dancing and bicycling and other activities. So they focused on the woman's market by highlighting exercise charts for running, walking, rope skipping, stair climbing, swimming, cycling, and stationary cycling.[13]

The Coopers recommended twenty-four points per week as a minimum number necessary to produce and maintain a satisfactory level of cardiovascular fitness for women.

THE AEROBICS WAY

Dr. Cooper's fourth book on aerobic exercise was called *The Aerobics Way.** The book is an update of his "aerobics system." Here, Cooper assails his critics and presents some facts and figures to support his system, a system he feels is an effective means of becoming fit and reducing selected coronary heart disease risk factors.

In *The Aerobics Way* the point system is updated, new fitness tests are presented to determine your fitness level (walking, swimming, and bicycling), and Cooper is more specific about fitness problems and how to deal with them. Although the system is the same as his three other books, *The Aerobics Way* is Cooper's best effort. He has more data, he plays down the fitness test at the outset of the program, and he provides programs for patients who have undergone coronary bypass surgery. He is much more conservative than in the first three books, a step that should make some of his physician critics happy.

The only criticism is the by-the-numbers approach. *The Aerobics Way* is well researched, backed with facts, and easy to understand. Beginning people in fitness will find this book most helpful. The experienced aerobic enthusiast will like the new facts.

CRITICISMS

Despite the popularity of *Aerobics, The New Aerobics,* and *Aerobics for Women—Aerobics* having over six million copies sold and at least fifteen translations [14]—Cooper has not been without critics. Some have had extremely harsh words to say about his plan. A Dallas cardiologist complains, "He's a

* K. H. Cooper, *The Aerobics Way.* NY: M. Evans, 1977.

publicity hound who hires a few doctors to work for him and goes around the country screaming that he can rescue everybody by running them!" [15] Some physicians contend that Cooper may be encouraging people to exercise who shouldn't, and they disapprove of his flamboyant personal style, which they feel is a violation of the medical profession's prohibition against self-promotion.[16]

Doctors Meyer Friedman, M.D., and Ray H. Rosenman, M.D., co-authors of the best seller *Type A Behavior and Your Heart,* agree that exercise does indeed enhance "the vigor of the heart muscle and its subjection to nervous control," but add that this "has absolutely no bearing on the state of the coronary arteries." [17] Friedman has further explained that "what we're concerned about is whether the heart's arteries are free and open, and there's no evidence that running opens those arteries." [18]

Dr. George Sheehan, M.D., feels that Cooper did a super job on documenting the effects of exercise, but that he missed the point about exercise being enjoyable, referring to Cooper as "a by-the-numbers researcher . . ." [19]

Researchers at the University of Toronto found that Cooper had undervalued some sports—soccer and tennis, for example. They also found that "when equal durations of activity are compared, the energy expenditures needed to earn a given point score differ from one form of activity to another," and they proposed a modification of the point system to "take account of the known effects of intensity of effort, initial fitness, and frequency and duration of effort on the training process." [20] The study did note, however, that the "exact equivalence of the points awarded for different types of activity is not over important in a simple and popular system of training." [21]

Frank Vitale, Associate Supervisor of Physical Education at the University of California at San Diego, writes, "Important as aerobic activities are, they are still not the complete answer to physical fitness through exercise. Other elements or modes of fitness, such as flexibility and coordination, are needed at all ages." [22]

Dr. Laurence Morehouse agrees with Vitale's complaint that Cooper's emphasis on heart, circulation, and oxygen consumption resulted in neglect of some other important aspects of fitness. He laments the lack of attention to muscle development. Morehouse is also afraid that Cooper has misled his readers by not considering individual differences via pulse rate.[23]

Dr. Thomas K. Cureton, Ph.D., Professor Emeritus of Physical Education at the University of Illinois, has been the most vocal critic of Dr. Cooper's program. *Consumer Guide®* invited Dr. Cureton to bring us up to date on his side of the aerobics debate. He declined, preferring instead to send copies of past papers and statements, which he feels adequately represent his point of view. Cureton's major criticism of the aerobics plan centers on the emphasis Cooper places on intensity of exercise. He regards the devotion to charts, points, oxygen-use rate, distance covered, etc., as fanatic attention to detail, placing unnecessary pressure on the exerciser to strive toward a specific goal. In his opinion, the most important factor in cardiovascular fitness improvement and in reduction of blood lipids (fats) and body fat is the length of time an exercise is performed. Basing his convictions on thirty years of experience in fitness development at the University of Illinois, Dr. Cureton has concluded that forty-five minutes to one hour of any vigorous activity performed five or six times a week at a comfortable (not straining) pace will produce fitness benefits.[24]

Dr. Cureton also maintains that the *Aerobics* program "is certainly not suitable for older people. A mixed on-and-off program, slower, but longer to add up enough kilocalories, may be very successful." [25]

A graduate student of Dr. Cureton's, Dr. Sharon Plowman, Ph.D., conducted an experiment comparing Cureton's Continuous Rhythmical Exercise Program with that of Cooper's thirty-point system. Plowman and Cureton found that the Cureton exercise group improved significantly more than those on the aerobics program in all measures.[26]

REBUTTAL

Consumer Guide® asked Dr. Cooper to respond to these criticisms. His comments are summarized in five areas.

INTENSITY. Dr. Cooper points out that those who regard the aerobics program as too intense are forgetting that at least twenty-eight different exercises qualify for points in the aerobics system. Some are far less demanding than jogging, which is one of the most intense. Low-intensity exercises such as walking must be of longer duration, but they are effective. With this approach, Cooper is convinced that nearly anyone, regardless of medical condition (with medical evaluation and supervision) can effectively enter his program.

CORONARY HEART DISEASE. In response to Dr. Friedman's statement that running doesn't open arteries, Cooper makes clear that he knows of nothing that will open up clogged arteries. He seriously doubts that atherosclerosis can be reversed even through diet. He looks to exercise as an aid in improving collateral circulation, oxygen utilization at the tissue level, extraction of the oxygen in the blood being pumped from the heart, and efficiency of the heart.

THE POINT SYSTEM. Cooper thinks the point system has been the key to the success of the aerobics concept in that, regardless of what critics say, people are basically goal-oriented. Studies have shown that most people who reach the "good" category of fitness were averaging thirty-four aerobics points per week and those in the "excellent" classification of fitness were averaging fifty. Even though many were not joggers, they participated regularly in other types of physical activity to the extent that they achieved the necessary points.[27]

Dr. Cooper concedes that the points were probably too low for some sports. His most recent book, *The Aerobics Way,* includes considerable upgrading. Soccer, for example, which the Toronto group felt was undervalued, will probably be increased from six to nine points per hour. He adds that he and his colleagues are making an effort to measure as many as possible of the exercises for which he awards points, but that they will again have to rely in some cases on literature documenting energy cost for various activities. They have from time to time found inaccuracies in this literature but will use such sources until new studies can be done.

NARROW FOCUS. Dr. Cooper claims that the statement that aerobics overlooks other components of fitness is not accurate. The aerobics program includes warm-up calisthenics, a mandatory cool-down, and the conditioning calisthenics or weight lifting. He himself engages in calisthenics and weight lifting regularly—after the aerobics workout. The program was designed *primarily* to counteract the cardiovascular/pulmonary problems; musculoskeletal conditioning and figure contouring do assume a secondary role.

EMPHASIS ON NUMBERS. Finally, Cooper accepts George Sheehan's "fitness by number" label: "I have indeed developed a system of 'fitness by the numbers,' but I think the concept is a good one," he explained. "I am trying to study exercise and determine its value in a very scientific fashion. Unless there is some way to measure the physical activity in a fairly simple, reliable form, it will not be possible to achieve this goal. If Dr. Sheehan has a better way to quantify accurately the values of exercise in the prevention and rehabilitation of disease, I would be delighted to hear his recommendations."

SUMMING UP

Because of the popularity of Cooper's program and the number of criticisms lodged against it, *Consumer Guide®* asked another expert to evaluate the aerobics program. Dr. Paul Ribisl, Ph.D., associate professor of physical education at Wake Forest University, a respected fitness authority and researcher and an active member of the American College of Sports Medicine, agreed to comment.

Dr. Ribisl agrees with Cooper that the aerobics system allows a wide range of activities of varying intensities and should not be faulted as overemphasizing intensity. "Moreover," says Ribisl, "he provides a starter program of six weeks or so to gradually introduce people to the exercise."

Cooper does place a great deal of emphasis on the timing of exercise, which can push some people to overdo it. *Consumer Guide®* would prefer to see an individual participate for the joy of activity rather than to achieve extra points. But it is true that many people are goal-oriented. To be sure you are not overextending yourself, you should check your pulse rate periodically to make sure you do not exceed the 70 percent to 85 percent range, a precaution suggested by Frank Vitale: "The check may very well indicate that you should spend a longer time at a particular level than that shown on the training charts. It can serve, then, as a valuable safety device as well as a method of providing greater flexibility." [28]

Dr. Ribisl does not share Cooper's belief that exercise will improve collateral circulation. He says instead, "The real benefit of exercise comes from helping people tolerate progressively greater loads during exercise. The research has yet to document any reversal in the buildup of deposits within the arteries through either exercise or diet. What will happen is that the skeletal muscles will be able to do more and more work and make the person more efficient so that there is less demand on the heart."

Consumer Guide® agrees that the status of exercise in preventing coronary artery disease is still unknown. The research has not been definitive. Cooper, of course, believes that it will be proved that exercise helps prevent heart disease. Moreover, he recognizes that the average sedentary person can't wait a hundred years for research to prove that exercise helps prevent heart disease. He is persuaded by his own research and that of others that people who engage in cardiovascular exercise reduce the number of coronary heart disease risk factors.[29]

A serious oversight in the first book *(Aerobics)* was Cooper's casual approach to a physical checkup prior to engaging in the exercise program and taking the 12-Minute Run. He did correct this omission in subsequent books and editions.

The Cooper/Cureton debate is distressing. Both highly respected in the fitness field and both thoroughly familiar with the literature and research in this area, they have strikingly similar goals and priorities. As Ribisl points out,

Cooper, of course, places a greater *emphasis* on cardio-respiratory fitness, while Cureton places his *emphasis* not only on the cardio-respiratory aspect of fitness but on total fitness, which includes flexibility, muscle strength, and endurance as well. Moreover, Cooper tends to emphasize intensity more than Cureton; Cureton looks at total work as the key. Another point to note is that Cureton's program seems to work best in a group setting such as a Y, while Cooper's program is more suitable to an individual setting. But both are by and large trying to achieve the same end.

Consumer Guide® questions the studies comparing Cooper's program with those of others, particularly Cureton's Continuous Rhythmical Exercise Program. A close look at the design of the studies shows that the investigation was biased in favor of the Continuous Rhythmical Exercise group in that this group did a greater amount of exercise and did it more frequently than did the Cooper group. Furthermore, according to Dr. Ribisl, a close look at the data shows that there was no significant difference between the groups with respect to their gains in the 12-Minute Run. He concluded (and *Consumer Guide®* concurs) that the exercise testing set-up was not quite fair since a bicycle test was used to evaluate the effects of a running program.

The charge that aerobics is not a total fitness program is somewhat justified. Cooper undervalues calisthenics and is vague in recommending strength-building and flexibility exercises.

Another problem is that Cooper recommends different minimum amounts of exercise for men and women (thirty and twenty-four points respectively). Cooper justifies this position by stating "that most women's total aerobic capacity is smaller than most men's" because of their smaller size. He feels his research indicates a woman needs only twenty-four points to achieve a good fitness level.[30] *Consumer Guide®* feels that there is no need to differentiate between men and women.

Consumer Guide® Rating: The aerobics programs outlined by Dr. Cooper are by far the easiest programs to implement for the on-your-own cardiovascular exerciser. The charts are easy to follow. The charts are interesting and fun because you can make comparisons between activities with respect to their cardiovascular worth. In *The New Aerobics, Aerobics for Women,* and *The Aerobics Way,* he provides good guidelines and procedures to follow before engaging in exercise. He recommends a starter program. And whether the experts like it or not, he does give people a goal they can work toward, which many seem to need. Although it is still too early to say that twenty-four to thirty points a week is a desirable level of activity, the system fairly well meets the standards set forth by the American College of Sports Medicine and the American Heart Association. *Consumer Guide®* feels, though, that Cooper should have included some specific recommendations regarding flexibility and strength-building exercises.

In *Aerobics,* the two major faults were (1) the failure to clearly require the physical checkup prior to starting the program and (2) too great an emphasis on the 12-Minute Run. The later books corrected these flaws.

The New Aerobics, Aerobics for Women, and *The Aerobics Way* are rated as excellent, and *Aerobics* as good.

WALKING AND JOGGING YOUR WAY TO FITNESS

The earliest and most natural forms of exercise are walking and running. Primitive human beings survived by being able to walk or jog great distances.

But times have changed. We still have the body that was designed to cover twenty-five or more miles a day, but today it rebels as soon as we attempt a thirty-minute walk, let alone a fifteen-minute jog. We Americans marvel at the stamina of the Tarahumara Indians of Mexico, who race at high altitudes in kickball games and relays that often last up to two days and cover one hundred to two hundred miles. Perhaps our fascination with walking and jogging programs is a subconscious recognition of our natural bent toward this kind of activity. Dr. Thaddeus Kostrubala, M.D., chief of psychiatry at Mercy Hospital in San Diego, believes that running has an anthropological basis: "For three million years genus *Homo* had to run to survive. Our femur [thighbone] is designed for running. Imposition of the city, only 1/600th of our history, made man a fixed animal, and heart disease followed. Part of the well-being we experience in running I believe to be a return to our basic nature. We are resonating with our heritage." [31]

Walking and jogging programs are very popular today and definitely deserve attention in any evaluation of fitness programs in modern-day America.

JOHNSON AND BASS: CREATIVE WALKING FOR PHYSICAL FITNESS.

In *Creative Walking for Physical Fitness,* Harry Johnson, M.D., and Ralph Bass present the thesis that walking is perfect for achieving physical fitness. According to Johnson, former medical director of the Life Extension Institute, walking is beneficial to cardiovascular health, weight control, figure control, mental activity, and overall health.[32]

A men's program recommends walking every day. (Figure 12 presents two sample weeks.) A second walking program was established for women because Dr. Johnson believed that most women would not be able to keep up with the plan outlined for men. He acknowledged that women need exercise as much as men do and should also adopt a regular schedule, but states that the difference in physical makeup must be taken into account:

> Obviously, she is not as strong as a man; her bones are smaller and lighter and she is, overall, less muscular. Moreover, since she is not usually as tall as a man, her stride is apt to be shorter. Finally, the structure of her pelvis differs from that of a man, resulting in greater pelvic rotation as she walks. This can be a source of some additional fatigue over the course of a lengthy walk.[33]

Johnson allows that a woman may find she can get up to three and a half miles an hour comfortably and should feel free to adopt this pace if she enjoys it. "However, our plan calls for the slower pace, and the plan covers a period of nine weeks instead of the ten weeks of the man's program. At the end of the nine-week period, the woman walker should have settled comfortably into a routine that she can stay with indefinitely."[34]

FIGURE 12 / SAMPLE CREATIVE WALKING PLAN FOR MEN

WEEK 1

During this week, try to keep to level ground. Stay within the recommended distances, even though you may feel you can do more.

Day 1	Walk 1 mile	slow (3 mph)
Day 2	Repeat Day 1	
Day 3	Walk 1½ miles	slow (3 mph)
Day 4	Repeat Day 3	
Day 5	Walk 2 miles	slow (3 mph)
Day 6	Repeat Day 5	
Day 7	Walk 2½ miles	slow (3 mph)

WEEK 9

You should now be in condition to undertake longer walks, perhaps hikes in the countryside up to ten miles or more on all kinds of terrain. A Saturday or Sunday is the most suitable day, of course, in the case of an employed person.

Day 1	Walk 8 miles	moderate (4 mph)
Day 2	Repeat Day 1	
Day 3	Walk 8½ miles	moderate (4 mph)
Day 4	Repeat Day 3	
Day 5	Walk 9 miles	moderate (4 mph)
Day 6	Repeat Day 5	
Day 7	Walk up to 10 miles	moderate (4 mph)

H. Johnson and R. Bass, *Creative Walking for Physical Fitness*. NY: Grosset and Dunlap, 1970, pp. 24 and 28, pp. 34 and 37.

Consumer Guide® Rating: *Creative Walking for Physical Fitness* is a marginal fitness program. The idea is sound; walking has clearly been shown to be one way to improve cardiovascular fitness and attain better body composition, and it does permit the heart rate to reach proper target heart

SAMPLE CREATIVE WALKING PLAN FOR WOMEN

WEEK 1

As in the man's program, do not attempt rough or hilly country walking this first week. And make haste slowly.

Day 1	Walk 880 yds. (1½ mile)	slow (3 mph)
Day 2	Repeat Day 1	
Day 3	Walk 1760 yds. (1 mile)	slow (3 mph)
Day 4	Repeat Day 3	
Day 5	Walk 1½ miles	slow (3 mph)
Day 6	Repeat Day 5	
Day 7	Walk 2 miles	slow (3 mph)

WEEK 8

Day 1	Walk 4½ miles	slow (3mph)
Day 2	Repeat Day 1	
Day 3	Walk 5 miles	slow (3mph)
Day 4	Repeat Day 3	
Day 5	Walk 5½ miles	slow (3mph)
Day 6	Repeat Day 5	
Day 7	Walk 6 miles	slow (3 mph)

rate ranges (60 percent to 90 percent).[35] The problem is that Dr. Johnson outlines a walking program that doesn't "make haste slowly." For the fit, a goal of eight to ten miles a day after nine weeks of training may be acceptable, but for the average (unfit) American, *Creative Walking* asks far too much too soon. The speed of walking (three to four mph) is satisfactory, and so is the idea of breaking the distance up into several walks a day. But asking people to walk two and a half miles a day at the end of the first week and five and a half miles a day after three weeks is a big order. Logic and research indicate that more time should be spent acquainting the exercisers with walking.[36] Furthermore, walking elicits high pulse rates in the unfit, and it would therefore seem unnecessary to exceed thirty minutes or so of exercise in the initial stages.

Distance training such as that outlined by Johnson can also bring about orthopedic problems. Too much distance, even if only walking, may cause leg problems for the unfit or for the person who walks incorrectly. (A more complete discussion of this problem will be found in the evaluation of jogging.)

Dr. Johnson also treads dangerous ground in recommending separate programs for men and women. Chapter 5 described research that indicates that there is no need to devise different plans for men and women.

This evaluation of "marginal" is unfortunate, for walking can be enjoyed by practically everyone, and there is some valuable information in *Creative Walking*. Johnson provides sound insight into the psychological benefits of walking, the importance of consulting your doctor, and other topics. But the program is just too ambitious. Walking is an excellent activity for physical fitness but not in the manner outlined by Dr. Johnson.

BOWERMAN AND HARRIS: JOGGING

The use of jogging (light running and walking) for physical conditioning originated with Arthur Lydiard, the New Zealand Olympic track coach. When some of his runners were ready to retire from competition but expressed a desire to retain their high level of fitness, Lydiard developed a jogging program to meet their needs. Because of his training regimens and enthusiasm, jogging is now a popular pastime in New Zealand.

In 1962, Bill Bowerman, the coach of the University of Oregon's track team, toured New Zealand and noticed the great number of jogging clubs and the zest of New Zealanders. Feeling his own fitness was not up to par, he decided to do something about it. On his return to the United States, he began to jog regularly. And he asked himself, "Why couldn't the same principles, in scaled-down versions, be applied to train typical businessmen and housewives in poor physical condition from lack of exercise?" [37]

The result was *Jogging,* published in 1967, in which Bowerman and W. E. Harris explained the hows and whys of jogging. Dr. Harris, a cardiologist, was especially interested in the role of regular exercise in decreasing the risk of heart disease. The two conducted studies of adults aged twenty-five to sixty-six. Their findings were positive and impressive, and again the news found a ready audience.

In the book, the authors outlined three twelve-week schedules. Plan A is for men and women in less than average physical condition (a totally sedentary person, a person recovering from an accident or illness, or an obese person more than 20 percent above desired weight. Plan B is for men and women in average condition (able to do normal chores and play occasional golf). Plan C is for men and women in better-than-average physical condition (very active people—hunters, skiers, fishers, and people who engage in outdoor or other strenuous sports). A few sample schedules from Plan A are presented in Figure 13.

Plan B is similar to Plan A except that one mile is covered in the first week, and two and a half miles during Week 12. The jog sequences are longer in Plan B. Plan C is an advancement of Plan B. The distance covered the first week is one and a quarter miles; after twelve weeks, four to five miles.

THE JOGGING CONTROVERSY

Criticisms of jogging are directed not so much at the Bowerman and Harris book as against the principle of jogging as a means of achieving physical fitness. Criticisms have come from both the medical profession and the public press. *Consumer Guide*® here focuses on those considered most legitimate and those that have attracted most attention.

FIGURE 13 / SAMPLE BOWERMAN AND HARRIS
Jogging CHARTS

PLAN A

WEEK 1

Pace 1 = 110 yds. at 55 to 60 seconds, or 25 to 30 seconds for 55 yds.

Monday			Pace
(total distance: ½ mile using the following pattern)			
(1) Jog 55 yds.	Walk 55 yds.	4 times	1
(2) Jog 110 yds.	Walk 110 yds.		1
(3) Jog 55 yds.	Walk 55 yds.	2 times	1

Tuesday 5- to 10-minute walk; easy stretching exercises
Wednesday

(total distance: ½ mile using the following pattern)			
(1) Jog 55 yds.	Walk 55 yds.	4 times	1
(2) Jog 110 yds.	Walk 110 yds.		1
(3) Jog 55 yds.	Walk 55 yds.	2 times	1

Thursday 5- to 10-minute walk; easy stretching exercises
Friday

(total distance: ½ mile using the following pattern)			
(1) Jog 55 yds.	Walk 55 yds.	4 times	1
(2) Jog 110 yds.	Walk 110 yds.		1
(3) Jog 55 yds.	Walk 55 yds.	2 times	1

Saturday 5- to 10-minute walk; change the scenery
Sunday 5- to 10-minute walk; easy stretching exercises

WEEK 12

Pace 3 = 110 yds. at 35 to 40 seconds
Pace 4 = 110 yds. at 25 to 30 seconds

Monday Pace
(total distance: 1½ miles using the following pattern)

(1)	Jog 110 yds.	Walk 110 yds.		3 or 4
(2)	Jog 220 yds.	Walk 110 yds.	2 times	3 or 4
(3)	Jog 330 yds.	Walk 110 yds.	3 times	3 or 4
(4)	Jog 110 yds.	Walk 110 yds.	2 times	3 or 4

Tuesday 5- to 10-minute walk; easy stretching exercises

Wednesday
(total distance: 1½ miles using the following pattern)

(1)	Jog 110 yds.	Walk 110 yds.	2 times	3 or 4
(2)	Jog one half mile in 10 to 12 minutes; walk and repeat.			
(3)	Jog 110 yds.	Walk 110 yds.	2 times	3 or 4

Thursday 5- to 10-minute walk; easy stretching exercises

Friday
(total distance: 1½ miles using the following pattern)

(1)	Jog 110 yds.	Walk 110 yds.	2 times	3 or 4
(2)	Jog 330 yds.	Walk 110 yds.		3 or 4
(3)	Slow jog for 4 to 6 minutes			
(4)	Jog 110 yds.	Walk 110 yds.	2 times	3 or 4

Saturday
Consider optional

Sunday
Optional program or 10-minute walk; stretching exercises

Modified and adapted from: W. J. Bowerman and W. E. Harris, *Jogging.* NY: Grosset and Dunlap, 1967, pp. 45 and 67.

ORTHOPEDIC. A jogger's foot hits the ground 600 to 750 times during each mile covered. That's rough treatment, especially if the running is done on a hard surface. The problem is compounded if the runner uses an inappropriate shoe ("tennies" are not running shoes!). When a shoe lacks support, the arch can flatten and injuries can occur throughout the lower extremities, from the foot to the hip. Even the back may be involved.

Physicians report that typical injuries include shin splints (pain along the inside of the shin),[38] stress fractures to the bones of the lower leg and foot, [39] Achilles tendinitis (tearing and inflammation of the tendon of the calf),[40] plantar fasciitis (tearing of tissue near or bruising of the heel bone),[41] and chondromalacia (a knee ailment).[42] *Runner's World* polled its readers and reported much the same list of common injuries: "knees (22 percent of the runners), Achilles tendons (20 percent), shin splints (10 percent), forefoot strain and fracture (9 percent), heels (7 percent), aches (7 percent)." [43] It is the current consensus among experts who practice sports medicine *and* run or jog that most of the injuries are due to overwork, faulty shoes, weakness and lack of flexibility, and improper running techniques.[44]

Dr. George A. Sheehan, M.D., has called attention to a related problem; running causes a loss of flexibility in the back of the legs, and a loss of strength of the muscles on the shin as opposed to those on the calf and of the stomach muscles compared to the back. Because of the lack of flexibility, exercises that stretch the muscles in the back of the legs (upper and lower) and lower back are necessary. Strength-building exercises for the muscles of the shin and the abdomen must also be incorporated.[45]

The orthopedic considerations are valid. Jogging can produce certain ailments in susceptible individuals. The key to avoiding these ailments is to take a number of precautions: be careful about the type of surface you run on; select high-quality running shoes; perform stretching exercises to counteract the lack of flexibility; and improve the muscle strength of major muscle groups.

CARDIOVASCULAR. There is considerable disagreement over the effect of jogging on the heart. Some of the experts are convinced that such exercise does no particular good; others believe it can actually be dangerous.

Meyer Friedman and Ray H. Rosenman write in *Type A Behavior and Your Heart,* "There is no good solid evidence that physical indolence leads to coronary artery disease or that physical activity protects against the same disorder.... If you suffer from one of the certain causes of coronary artery disease or if you possess a Type A Behavior Pattern (a hostile, time-oriented, tense person), any real faith in the prophylactic potential of physical activity might be dangerously illusionary."[46] Friedman is strongly opposed to jogging on medical grounds and clearly feels that the jogging itself may be a risk: "If all joggers could be assured of a standby defibrillator [a machine that electronically restarts heartbeat] and someone trained to use it who could be at the scene within thirty seconds, I might even grow to love jogging."[47]

Other physicians agree that jogging is too vigorous and will cause or precipitate heart attacks. One of the most strongly worded examples of this point of view was the 1976 *Playboy* magazine article "Jogging Can Kill You." In the article, E. G. Schmidt, a physician, claimed that jogging can cause heart attacks, all sorts of leg and back problems, sagging breasts, and displaced ovaries.[48]

Still others such as Peter Steincrohn, M.D., think such vigorous activity is a waste of our limited supply of energy: "We were given somewhere between 2 and 2.5 billion heartbeats in our bank when we were born.... People who are born with weak hearts and with a smaller heartbeat bank should always take things easier. But even when born healthy, we can't afford to throw away and waste heartbeats by overexertion. You can't get back a wasted heartbeat."[49] This currently is the opinion of a very small number of doctors—yoga practitioners in particular.

Kenneth H. Cooper, M.D., a strong advocate of jogging, notes that:

> Our studies show a beautiful relationship between levels of physical fitness and a lowering of such things as blood glucose, blood triglycerides, cholesterol, body weight, percent of body fat, and blood pressure. We have shown a perfect relationship

between the levels of fitness and resting heart rate, pulmonary volume, and even levels of uric acid. We have been able to show in large studies of about 3,000 men that as they move up from very poor, poor, and fair to excellent category of fitness, their risk factors move down almost in a straight line relationship. For the first time we are showing the relationship between levels of fitness and selected coronary risk factors.[50]

And, according to Cooper, a real advantage of running is that, although the changes may occur with any type of activity that is of continuous nature (walking, swimming, cycling, etc.), running is especially valuable because you get the most benefit in the shortest period of time. Furthermore, little equipment is needed, and it is accessible and possible for almost everybody.

Dr. Thomas Bassler, a pathologist from Inglewood, California, and a strong leader in the American Medical Joggers Association, asserts flatly that "running builds strong hearts. Many high-risk patients are flourishing in cardiac rehabilitation programs that emphasize slow long distance running. Running programs can not only extend the lives of cardiac patients, but also those suffering from atherosclerosis and lung and liver diseases, which account for two-thirds of all natural deaths." [51]

The *Playboy* attack on jogging warrants special attention because it was so widely read and so condemning. *Consumer Guide®* carefully analyzed the article and agrees with the rebuttal by Dr. James Skinner, Ph.D. Skinner concluded that the article was written by a person "with little or no scientific background or evidence to substantiate his overstated opinions." [52] In fact, it was strictly an opinion piece, as no scientific data were given. *Consumer Guide®* deplores an approach in which a physician uses his professional status to popularize misinformation.

The belief that you can't get back a wasted heartbeat is ridiculous. There is no evidence that a person has a "bank" of only 2 to 2.5 billion heartbeats in a lifetime. But even if this were true, the statement reveals ignorance of an important principle of exercise physiology. As you train, your resting heart rate drops; consequently, you save heartbeats. For example, let's assume that you have a resting heart rate of 80 beats. Let's also assume that you get your heart rate up to 150 beats every day for a half-hour. That's an extra 70 heartbeats per minute for a half-hour, which comes out to 2,100 extra heartbeats a day. However, because of the training, your resting heart rate will probably drop 10 to 20 beats (to 60 or 70 beats per minute). If it drops only 10 beats per minute, the lower rate over the remaining 23½ hours would amount to 14,100 fewer beats per day than before training. By expending an extra 2,100 or so beats a day, you save another 14,100. That's a net gain of 12,000 heartbeats. So even if the "fixed number of heartbeats" theory were true, it doesn't follow that regular exercise uses too many.

MENTAL CONSIDERATIONS: "IT'S BORING." Many people criticize jogging as boring. Friedman and Rosenman voice this complaint. "Chug-chug-chugging along, looking neither to the right nor left, panting, the 'machine man' chugs along. And what is 'its' goal? To see if 'it' can chug-chug faster today than yesterday. And what is 'its' only joy? The soothing miraculous feeling of *relief* when the chug-chugging is finished." [53] Even Glenn Swengros, the former program director for the President's Council on Physical Fitness and Sports, used to say, "If jogging isn't the most boring thing around, it is right there in second place."

The mental argument is a tough one. Jogging is not for everyone. Some people do not have the body type or the inclination to run.[54] But to call it "boring" is not fair. Some people do like to run. Perhaps to Dr. Friedman it is "chug-chug-chugging," but to the jogging enthusiast this is not the case. Many people enjoy running a great deal. In fact, several psychiatrists and psychologists are using jogging as part of therapy programs to reduce anxiety and depression.[55]

Some experts feel that running can reduce Type A (tense, overstressed) behavior patterns. Dr. Joan Ullyot says, "I think that, approached as a relaxing, enjoyable pastime, as it should be, running is very relaxing and conducive to Type B [more relaxed, less time-oriented] personality habits." [56] Dr. Ronald M. Lawrence, M.D., founder and president of the American Medical Jogging Association, is even more dramatic in his enthusiasm: "Running is addictive. . . . It changes your whole life-style. Nobody's ever the same again. Running produces tranquillity. We know it changes a Type A personality into a Type B. You get away from the rat race on a regular basis." [57]

Consumer Guide® Rating: The Bowerman and Harris book provides an excellent program. It is slow, progressive, and allows for individual differences. It contains good advice on how to exercise ("train, don't strain"), and the progression includes work on stretching. (Unfortunately, no specific flexibility exercises are given for the legs and low back.) No outlandish claims are made.

The major drawback of the book is its regimented approach. The distances are based on a quarter-mile track, and the times are quite specific. The training schedules read like a training schedule for track competition. The program is obviously limited to one primary activity—jogging—and suffers from a perhaps natural tendency to ignore the value of other activities. Finally, no strength-building exercises are given.

CURTIS MITCHELL: THE JOY OF JOGGING

The Joy of Jogging, written by science/health writer Curtis Mitchell,[58] describes one man's experience with jogging—his initial cynicism toward exercising, his need (angina pain), his acceptance, and finally his evangelical zeal. It is a book that presents some homespun physiology and some conclusions based on the opinion of experts.

Mitchell's program is similar to the one presented in *Jogging*. He provides a thirteen-week beginners' program, a thirteen-week intermediate plan, and a thirteen-week advanced plan. Figure 14 presents three sample weeks of the thirteen-week beginners' plan.

FIGURE 14   /   SAMPLE *Joy of Jogging* BEGINNERS' PLAN

1st week: Warm-up and calisthenics. 15 minutes.
               Walk one mile each exercise day.
7th week: Warm-up and calisthenics.
               Walk one mile.
               Walk-jog one mile.
               Walk one mile.
               Walk-jog one mile.
13th week: Warm-up and calisthenics.
               Walk-jog four miles.

C. Mitchell, *The Joy of Jogging*. NY: Rutledge Books and Ace News Company, 1968, pp. 78–79.

The thirteen-week intermediate plan is simply an extension of the beginners' plan, and the advanced plan recommends that you continue as before,

> ... but jog three or four miles continuously at least three and, if possible, five days every week. Six months of jogging are behind you. Your heart is renewed, your feet and legs are toughened, your mind is unafraid of pain or labored breathing.
>
> Now, if you want to compete with yourself you can try what the track buffs call interval training. It is exactly like walk-jog training except you jog-*sprint*.[59]

There are four major differences between Bowerman's and Harris's *Jogging* and Mitchell's *Joy of Jogging*. First, Mitchell recommends fifteen minutes of warm-up and Bowerman and Harris about five minutes. Second, Mitchell has you walk-jog four miles after thirteen weeks, Bowerman and Harris about one and a half miles. Bowerman and Harris don't recommend four miles until about Week 7 of Chart 3; that's after thirty-one weeks of training. Third, Bowerman and Harris are much more specific than Mitchell on distance and pace. Mitchell places more emphasis on distance. Finally, Mitchell recommends a jog-sprint at the advanced level, which Bowerman and Harris do not recommend at all.

Consumer Guide® Rating: *Consumer Guide*® rates *The Joy of Jogging* as marginal. It's excellent for a person in good physical condition but too vigorous for the average person. The recommended four miles of jogging after only thirteen weeks of training, and the suggested jog-sprinting make this quite an ambitious program. We cannot share Mitchell's confidence in the wisdom of such a strenuous program.

PRESIDENT'S COUNCIL ON PHYSICAL FITNESS AND SPORTS: JOGGING/RUNNING GUIDELINES

The President's Council on Physical Fitness and Sports has provided jogging/running guidelines for adults and children, including advice regarding medical clearance, clothing, shoes, how, when, and where.[60] The program is clear-cut, beginning with at least three times per week every other day. "If the beginner jogs every day, the chances of foot or leg problems developing are greater than if he jogs every other day. After the bones, ligaments, and muscles of the legs get used to supporting body weight while jogging, then a daily program can be developed." [61] On the days you don't jog, you are asked to perform stretching exercises or calisthenics, walk, or swim. The jogger is cautioned always to start each workout with a warm-up (a walk and stretching exercises) and end with tapering off in a walk. "Once the basic sixteen-week program is completed, a person should be experienced enough to design a regular exercise program to fit his own needs, schedule, facilities, and interests. Remember, the important thing is to exercise regularly—that is, every day or every other day." [62]

Consumer Guide® Rating: These guidelines constitute an excellent program, although similar to Bowerman and Harris in its somewhat regimented approach.

THE 2100 EXERCISE PLAN

The 2100 Program is found in *Live Longer Now,* a book written by John N. Leonard, J. L. Hofer, and N. Pritikin.[63] The key element is "roving." The authors claim that roving is the most natural of all exercises and may consist of walking, jogging, or running, or any variation or combination of these. "The key in roving is to set yourself a distance goal of so many miles. Then four or five times each week you set out to walk (or run, if you prefer) that distance. Enjoy yourself as you go. Go different places on different days if you like. Change the scenery whenever you want to." [64]

The plan, presented in Figure 15, is simple enough.

FIGURE 15 / THE 2100 PROGRAM
*The Ten Fundamental Principles of Exercise
Utilizing the Concept of Roving*

1 / Distance is important; time is not.
2 / Select a distance suited to yourself (see guidelines below).
3 / Rove your distance four or five times per week.
4 / As warm-up, begin each rove at a slow pace. That is all the warm-up needed.
5 / Increase your roving distance only when you are ready.
6 / Use your heart recovery test (below) as your gauge to slow down or speed up.
7 / Give yourself variety.

8 / Do not strain or compete against the clock or against people.

9 / Always enjoy your roving.

10 / The program is for everyone: young or old, male or female.

Easy? The above is the only exercise listing you will ever see in the 2100 Exercise Program. This is all there is to it.

Rules for Selecting Your Distance:

1 / A few blocks if you are or have been very ill.

2 / 1½ miles if you are healthy but in poor-to-average condition.

3 / 3 miles if you are healthy and in good condition.

4 / 6 to 10 miles if you are healthy and in excellent condition.

Heart Recovery Test: *

1 / After a rove, stop and rest 60 seconds.

2 / Count your pulse (by feeling your wrist or your throat) over a 30-second time period.

3 / If this 30-second count exceeds 65, slow down on subsequent roves.

4 / When you are fully conditioned, your 30-second count will be near 50, even under conditions of heavy exercise.

* An adaptation of the internationally used Harvard Step Test.

J. L. Leonard, J. L. Hofer, and N. Pritikin, *Live Longer Now*. NY: Grosset and Dunlap, 1974, pp. 182–183.

Consumer Guide® Rating: A marginal-to-good cardiovascular program, the 2100 Exercise Plan possesses two flaws. The first is that the authors do not indicate what is meant by poor, average, good, or excellent condition. Second, the distances recommended in the excellent and poor categories (depending, of course, on what is meant by poor) might be excessive from an orthopedic point of view. For those in poor physical condition, one mile may be sufficient. For those in excellent condition, six to ten miles during the first few weeks may be traumatic to the lower extremities until they are conditioned to roving. If you are used to walking, running, or jogging six to ten miles, the program is acceptable. But if three miles a day has been your maximum, a sudden jump of three to seven more miles (regardless of the time) is excessive. A rule of thumb: When you are able to rove fifteen to twenty miles a week comfortably, *add one mile a week* running or jogging or two miles a week walking (a pulse check is O.K. for cardiovascular stress, but it does not tell you about your legs).

Consumer Guide® does, however, like the ideas of not using the clock and of relying on the pulse rate to see how well you have recovered from the exercise.

9

PULSE-RATED CARDIOVASCULAR EXERCISE PLANS

UNTIL PULSE-RATED EXERCISE CAME ALONG, EXERCISE WAS measured in time, distance, physical load, or number of actions performed. There was no way to measure one important missing element: effort.

Effort and work are not synonymous. Two people may run one mile up a 5-percent grade in eight minutes, and both would be performing the same amount of activity. For one, however, the run may be effortless, whereas the other may find it requires a good bit of effort. If the one finding it an effort trains consistently, soon running the mile in eight minutes will not be as hard. He or she becomes more proficient and the effort is reduced.

Most fitness programs have not taken into account this difference between work and effort. Programs intended for popular use are necessarily ultraconservative in starting point and rates of progression in order to avoid risk for the unconditioned. Exercisers do not know when to increase the level of activity so that maximum fitness is attained. Furthermore, the state of your body varies from day to day.

Sickness, fatigue, and biorhythms all affect its ability to respond.

According to many experts, it takes a kind of computer to gauge how much activity is required for training results, and many believe that your heart can serve as that computer. By exercising at a specific heart rate, you maintain a constant level of effort. (Fatigue, heat, sickness, and other conditions are automatically accounted for in that at such times less effort is needed to raise the heart rate to a given level.)

This chapter focuses on pulse-rated programs that include only minimal amounts of calisthenics.

LAURENCE E. MOREHOUSE: TOTAL FITNESS

In 1975, Dr. Laurence E. Morehouse, Ph.D., professor of exercise physiology and founder of the Human Performance Laboratory at UCLA, shocked fitness enthusiasts and exercise physiologists of the world with his book *Total Fitness*. This book made some startling claims:

> If you haven't exercised once in the last twenty years, you are nonetheless just two hours away from good physical condition, relative to the condition you were in when you began. At the end of twelve hours, you will be in excellent shape by any standards. You will look and feel better. Your waist will be thinner, your hips and thighs firmer. And you will be permanently rid of many pounds of fat.[1]

These attractive claims were welcome news to many fitness-conscious Americans. The Morehouse plan was far less demanding than the other fitness programs that had received public attention.

Morehouse divides fitness into three levels:

MINIMUM MAINTENANCE. The first is minimum maintenance—"the irreducible minimum below which you're going to experience degradation of function and structure."[2] To achieve this level, you need only to incorporate five simple habits into your everyday life:

1 / Limber up by reaching arms, twisting trunk, bending waist, and turning trunk.
2 / Stand for a total of two hours during the day.
3 / Lift something unusually heavy for five seconds.
4 / Walk briskly for at least three minutes to stimulate your cardiovascular system.
5 / Burn up three hundred calories a day in physical activity.[3]

None of this calls for special exercise. The requirements can supposedly be satisfied by focusing on activities already in your daily routine. For example, "you can maintain your present muscle tone by lifting a small child once a day ... [or] a few bags of heavy groceries will achieve the same results. The load on your muscles provides them with 'minimum maintenance.' " [4]

The last of the five is the big one, says Morehouse. Burning up activity calories requires movements that increase your pulse rate above 100 beats per minute. Walking, lifting, carrying, climbing, sexual activity—any of these will do. You can obtain your activity calories by gardening, chopping wood, and the like. Morehouse strongly recommends walking, bicycling, running, swimming, golf, tennis, table tennis, and dancing. The exercise doesn't have to be done continuously. For example, to burn up 300 calories by walking, you would have to walk three miles; this could be distributed over various times of the day (as you shop, etc.) as long as the total is three miles.

There is an alternative to even these minimal activities. You can simply stretch, stand, lift, and move briskly throughout the day. Morehouse believes you will burn 300 extra calories in this way.

GENERAL FITNESS. The second level is general fitness, "which provides you with a safe margin of adaptation for change, including emergencies, and enables you to get through the day without an undue amount of fatigue." [5] For this level, Morehouse recommends his thirty-minute-a-week program. The exerciser progresses through three stages of eight weeks each. During the first eight weeks, a session (to be repeated three times per week) includes one minute of limbering up, four minutes of muscle building, and five minutes of any continuous activity that raises your heartbeat to 60 percent of maximum. For example, let's assume you are forty years old. Morehouse instructs you to estimate your maximum heart rate by subtracting your age from 220. In this hypothetical case, then, your maximum heart rate would be 180 (220 minus 40), and 60 percent of 180 is 108. Therefore, 108 is your training heart rate—or any forty-year-old's, according to Morehouse.

After spending eight weeks at this level, you are then ready for Step 2. Again, it lasts eight weeks. Morehouse prescribes one minute of limbering up, four minutes of muscle endurance training, and six minutes of pulse-rated exercise at a new training heart rate—70 percent of your maximum. For example, a forty-year-old person would subtract 40 from 220 again (180), but this time take 70 percent of the 180 to arrive at a target rate of 126. Morehouse cautions against going any higher at this stage.

Step 3 is the final stage of your fitness-building program. Here Morehouse recommends two parts: (1) two minutes of muscle-strength building and (2) eight minutes of pulse-rated exercise at 80 percent of maximum heart rate. At this level, the training rate for the forty-year-old would be 80 percent of 180, or 144.

Figure 16 summarizes the three stages of the Morehouse plan.

MAINTENANCE. After 24 weeks, you are ready for what Morehouse calls maintenance—"preparation for fairly strenuous recreational or occupational activity." [6] He provides three maintenance programs, summarized here in Figure 17.

FIGURE 16 / THE MOREHOUSE FITNESS-BUILDING PROGRAM

Step One: *Tissue rebuilding and cardiovascular reconditioning, first eight weeks.*

MINUTES	EXERCISE
0–1	Limbering warm-up: reach, twist, bend, turn
1–2	15–20 pushaways
2–3	Sit-backs held for 15–20 seconds
3–4	Repeat pushaways
4–5	Repeat sit-backs
5–10	Continuous lope at 60-percent pulse
	Cool-down stroll

Step Two: *Muscular endurance and cardiovascular reconditioning, second eight weeks.*

	Limbering warm-up
0–1	40–50 pushaways (fast)
1–2	Sit-backs held for 40–50 seconds each
2–3	Repeat pushaways
3–4	Repeat sit-backs
4–10	Endurance intervals (30-second lope intervals alternated with 30 seconds of active rest at 70-percent pulse)
	Cool-down stroll

Step Three: *Muscular strength and cardiovascular reconditioning, third eight weeks.*

	Limbering warm-up
0–2	Alternate 1–5 pushaways with sit-backs held 1–5 seconds
2–10	Sprint intervals (15-second lope intervals alternated with 15 seconds of active rest at 80-percent pulse)
	Cool-down stroll

L. Morehouse and L. Gross, *Total Fitness.* NY: Pocket Books, Inc., 1976, pp. 235–236.

FIGURE 17 / THE MOREHOUSE MAINTENANCE PROGRAM

A

MINUTES	EXERCISE
0–1	Limbering warm-up
1–1.5	5 strength pushaways
1.5–2	Strength sit-backs, held 5 seconds each
2–10	Endurance lope (continuous at 80-percent pulse)

B

MINUTES	EXERCISE
0–1	Limbering warm-up
1–2	20 expansion pushaways
2–3	Expansion sit-backs held 20 seconds each
3–10	Endurance intervals (30 seconds of rapid cardio-respiratory exercise alternated with 30 seconds of "active rest," such as walking or slow pedaling, for 7 minutes at 80-percent pulse)

C

MINUTES	EXERCISE
0–1	Limbering warm-up
1–3	50 endurance pushaways
3–5	Endurance sit-backs held 50 seconds each
5–10	Sprint intervals (15 seconds of rapid circulo-respiratory exercise alternated with 15 seconds of "active rest," for 5 minutes at 80-percent pulse)

L. Morehouse and L. Gross, *Total Fitness*. NY: Pocket Books, Inc., 1976, p. 237.

CRITICISMS

Total Fitness has had many critics. According to *The Physician and Sportsmedicine,* physiologists have almost unanimously raised strong objections to the unrealistic claims for such an easy program.[7] Herbert deVries, Ph.D., director of the University of Southern California Exercise Physiology Laboratory, claims that the program "runs counter to almost all existing data from published research." [8]

Doctors Jack Wilmore, Ph.D., and R. James Barnard, Ph.D., two highly respected exercise physiologists, have been the most vocal critics. They believe that Morehouse and his collaborator L. Gross have exploded some exercise myths but created some new ones. Morehouse's reliability is questioned: "Areas where research evidence exists in abundance are contradicted or totally ignored in favor of isolated case studies or personal experiences which have yet to be evaluated by the scientific community and published in respected scientific journals." [9]

Wilmore and Barnard also list several statements in the book that are confusing to the public, misleading, unfounded, and/or downright incorrect. The Morehouse claims they object to are the following:

1 / "You can achieve and maintain fitness in twice the amount of time you require to brush your teeth."

2 / "If you haven't exercised once in the last twenty years, you are nonetheless just two hours away from good physical condition relative to the condition you were in when you began. At the end of twelve hours, you will be in excellent shape by any standards."

3 / "Muscle recovers about six times faster than circulatory tissue."

4 / "Nearly 90 percent of the body is water."

5 / "A pulse rate above 120 borders on intensive exertion."

6 / "A pulse rate of 160 is rated as 'very, very heavy.' "

7 / "An inch of pinch means 40 pounds of fat in most adults."

Dr. Wilmore recognizes the program's attractions: "We'd all like to believe what Morehouse contends. Unfortunately, there are really no data available to substantiate his program." [10] Dr. Michael Pollock, Ph.D., agrees: "It is pretty well documented now that you probably have to get twenty to thirty minutes of sustained effort at 80 percent to 90 percent of maximum effort at least three days a week. There's no easy way. . . . Only if the person has been sedentary for some time is there much benefit. Otherwise there's only minimal improvement, no weight loss, no body fat loss, and only slight cardiovascular improvement." [11]

Casey Conrad, Executive Director of the President's Council on Physical Fitness, concurs and adds a further point: "Do you realize that we have over two hundred sophisticated researchers laboring in our universities to learn more about fitness and health? Larry [Morehouse] isn't even one of the principal researchers. To say that it might do you harm to sweat is really pitiful." [12]

Consumer Guide® objects to one other point which has been neglected by the critics. Morehouse states in his book, "At the end of twelve hours . . . you will be permanently rid of many pounds of fat." [13] *Consumer Guide®* regards this statement as irresponsible. Assuming that during each of the twelve hours 300 to 600 calories are used up, the total in twelve hours would be 3,600 to 7,200 calories. That's one or two pounds of fat. It's hard to understand how a scientist could call that "many pounds of fat."

REBUTTAL

Morehouse has undertaken a lively counteroffensive. He fights back, answering critics by saying that it all depends upon the degree of fitness sought: "A world class athlete cannot by my method achieve the fitness his performance requires. But a nonathlete with a relatively sedentary lifestyle can make remarkable advances in fitness with slight effort in brief periods." [14]

To Wilmore and Barnard he responds that the minimum

duration of effective exercise is not yet known.[15] In repeating his contention that less than ten minutes of exercise may be effective in producing cardiovascular fitness, he cites three studies that supposedly show that high-intensity exercise of approximately 80 percent of maximum heart rate percent (remember, he starts at 60 percent) of relatively short duration (five minutes) may be effective in conditioning the heart and lungs.[16]

Morehouse also points out that strength development takes less time—six to ten seconds for each muscular effort:

> Thus it is possible to combine the several essential elements—a short limbering warm-up; a few minutes of mass, strength, or endurance development of muscular weakness areas of the body; and up to eight minutes of heart-rated cardio-respiratory exercise—into a ten-minute-a-day, three-day-a-week program that conditions the nonathletic adult to live life more fully and have a modest reserve of strength and endurance for emergencies which is all the fitness, i.e., *Total Fitness,* one needs at a mild level of daily life activity. By keeping the session short, body heat storage is minimized, the exercise is not uncomfortable and countless people who are unwilling to engage in more severe programs are encouraged to develop life-sustaining fitness.[17]

Consumer Guide® Rating: Laurence Morehouse has certainly stirred up a hornet's nest in the fitness and exercise world. *Total Fitness* polarized fitness enthusiasts and professionals. *Consumer Guide®* joins the critics and recognizes five fundamental problem areas.

INADEQUATE CARDIOVASCULAR TRAINING. Morehouse's program does not meet the minimum requirements of cardiovascular fitness as determined by research and outlined earlier in this book. Although researchers are still divided on the minimum amount of exercise needed to achieve cardiovascular fitness, most agree that less than ten minutes is not adequate—especially at the level Morehouse suggests at the start (60 percent of maximum).

INSUFFICIENT RESEARCH. Morehouse's retort to Wilmore's and Barnard's charges is almost a comedy of errors. The first of the three studies he used for support—by Doctors Marilyn Flint, Ph.D., Barbara Drinkwater, Ph.D., and Steve Horvath, Ph.D.—was apparently misquoted. Dr. Drinkwater herself contradicted his use of the work: "Dr. Morehouse has completely misinterpreted the results of our study." [18] She says that their report simply does not suggest the conclusions Morehouse reached!

The second study Morehouse used for support was done by E. A. Harris and B. B. Porter in 1958. It stated that 80 percent of the maximum heart rate was needed, not 60 percent as Morehouse suggested.

The third reference was to his own research—hardly an unbiased survey. And even his own research was based on a pulse rate of 80-percent intensity, not 60 percent, at eight minutes' duration. Only at Step 3 does the program prescribe eight minutes at 80 percent of heart-rate maximum.

RELIANCE ON "DAILY ROUTINE." Morehouse recommends lifting a baby or a few sacks of groceries daily to meet strength requirements. Doctors Wilmore and Barnard take exception: "While these activities may prevent total loss of muscular strength in extremely weak individuals, e.g., bedridden, there's no evidence to support the claim that these activities will help maintain desirable levels of muscular strength in the 'unfit' population, no matter how low your standards." [19]

MISLEADING TIME REQUIREMENTS. *Consumer Guide®* also questions the inconsistencies in *Total Fitness* regarding the exercise time required. On the cover and in the text, the authors recommend ten minutes a day three times a week (for a total of thirty minutes a week). They seem to forget that in the "minimum maintenance" stage they also ask each person to burn an extra 300 calories a day. That's good advice. However, to burn up that many extra calories the average person would have to exercise thirty to forty-five minutes. So Morehouse is asking for ten minutes of exercise three times a week *plus* thirty to forty-five minutes extra a day. Morehouse himself overlooks this extra requirement, emphasizing instead the thirty-minute-a-week slogan.

OVERSIMPLIFYING TO POPULARIZE. Morehouse's attempt to motivate the general (nonathletic) public to exercise is a laudable goal. Unfortunately, his book sells the public short. Dr. Samuel Fox, M.D., an internationally respected cardiologist and fitness expert (former director of the U.S. Public Health Service Program of Heart Disease and Stroke Control), notes that "the major hazard to the Morehouse approach is that people will make the sacrifices he asks, and then they will not find their lives enhanced." [20]

People may *like* Morehouse's program and respond to the kind of punchy, confident promotion techniques that have been used to publicize it, but the catchy phrases fall short of the truth about exercising for fitness.

Total Fitness ranks as a poor program; *Consumer Guide*® finds it filled with many misleading, incorrect, and marginal statements. It has done a great disservice to the fitness movement.

LENORE R. ZOHMAN: BEYOND DIET

In 1974, Dr. Lenore R. Zohman's thirty-six-page booklet *Beyond Diet: Exercise Your Way to Fitness and Heart Health* was published by Mazola Corn Oil as a public service. Dr. Zohman, an internationally recognized physician and exercise physiologist, set out to provide a means to improve cardiovascular fitness, reduce selected coronary heart disease risk factors, and reduce body weight and fat.

She begins by recommending a physical checkup for sedentary prospective exercisers, with special attention to the cardiovascular system, blood pressure, muscles, and joints. The blood should be analyzed and a resting electrocardiogram taken. And "most importantly, the examination before starting an exercise program should include an exercise stress test." [21] Zohman provides some commonsense guidelines to follow in the event that such a test is not given in your area or your budget precludes it.

The program is based on target heart rates. Dr. Zohman recommends that normal people reach 70 percent to 85 percent of their maximum heart rate (based on age). She also suggests that to get the pulse rate up to that range the activity must be sustained—i.e., walking, jogging, running, swimming, cycling, rope skipping, etc.

The exercise program begins with five to ten minutes of warm-up, followed by twenty to thirty minutes of exercise at target-zone heart rate and five to ten minutes of cooling-down. The activity is to be performed at least three nonconsecutive days each week.

The booklet provides some simple guidelines on saturated versus unsaturated fats, danger signs of exercise, and tips on motivation and bicycling equipment. Dr. Zohman also explains how to count your pulse rate and discusses the relative merits of various exercises in inducing cardiovascular fitness.

Consumer Guide® Rating: An excellent program for cardiovascular fitness, the Zohman plan meets recommended guidelines for intensity (70 percent to 85 percent of maximum heart rate); duration (twenty to thirty minutes); and frequency (three nonconsecutive days a week). Furthermore, it includes a variety of activities, giving the individual ample opportunity to match the exercise to personal preference. The pulse-rate emphasis assures that age and physical condition variations will not be overlooked.

A few shortcomings should be noted. There is no discussion of flexibility or of muscle strength and endurance. And the Zohman recommendation of three exercise days per week falls short by one day of the four-day-per-week minimum that *Consumer Guide*® recommends for ideal body composition.

Overall, however, Dr. Zohman has done an excellent job in thirty-six pages.

M. F. GRAHAM: PRESCRIPTION FOR LIFE

Dr. M. F. Graham's *Prescription for Life* was the first of the pulse-rated exercise books available to the public. Dr. Graham, a pediatrician in Dallas, Texas, focuses on running in place, jogging, walking, cycling, or any activity that is sustained and gets the pulse rate into the desired range (approximately 140 beats per minute). The program consists of five steps:

1 / At a predetermined time of day, clad in clothing appropriate for the occasion, and in some place where you will not be disturbed, count your pulse rate while sitting and record in chart form. . . .

2 / Limber up with mild calisthenics. (Toe touches, knee bends, and trunk twists. Do only a few.)

3 / Start in-place running (running in one spot) at a slow "jog" pace (about two steps per second), and continue for two minutes. . . . A certain amount of breathlessness will be experienced by the untrained; unless it is extremely difficult to carry on, this initial breathlessness should be regarded as physiologic. It is essential. Do not at any time, however, force yourself to continue when you feel it is absolutely beyond your capacity for the time.

4 / *Immediately* after you stop running, sit down and check your pulse rate again and record alongside your pre-exercise pulse rate. . . .

5 / Continue sitting and check your pulse each minute after stopping exercise for three minutes, and again ten minutes after, and record. . . .[22]

These five steps are to be repeated on three different occasions—no more than a day apart and after you are well rested. After your pulse rates are recorded, you average each set—before exercise; immediately after; and two, three, and ten minutes after exercise. These five different average pulse rates are what Graham calls your minimum exercise response (MER).

The five pulse rates are to be measured each time you exercise. You are to limit yourself to two minutes of exercise until your MER satisfies Graham's "Five-Point Rule":

1 / The pulse rate one minute after exercise should not exceed 110 or thereabouts.

2 / The pulse rate two minutes after exercise should be at least ten beats per minute less than that one minute after exercise.

3 / The pulse rate three minutes after exercise should be at least ten beats per minute less than that two minutes after exercise.

4 / The pulse rate ten minutes after exercise should very nearly approximate the resting pulse rate, although here more variation is allowable with longer periods of exercise.

5 / Undue breathlessness should not persist for longer than two minutes.[23]

Every few days you are to increase the exercise time (running in place) by a minute or so until you are able to run for ten minutes. Then you are to begin to double-time your steps. When you are able to double-time at least five of the ten minutes of running in place, extend the duration of exercise and speed of running. This break-in period or conditioning period is crucial.

After the conditioning period, most people go outdoors and run, cycle, or swim. Strive to increase the running time to twenty-five to thirty minutes over a distance of about three miles. Your pulse rate should be at least 60 percent of its "capable range." (This is approximately the same as 70 percent to 85 percent of maximum. For example, a resting heart rate of 60 and a maximum of 180 equals 120 range. Sixty percent of 120 is 72. That added to the resting heart rate (60) is 132. A forty-year-old person would have a maximum of 180, and 70 percent of 180 is about 126 beats per minute.)

Consumer Guide® Rating: Dr. Graham's *Prescription for Life* is an excellent program. The book's major disadvantage is the narrow focus on running and running in place (with other activities considered only casually). Furthermore, no attention is paid to the importance of flexibility and muscle strength and endurance.

ROY ALD: JOGGING, AEROBICS AND DIET

Roy Ald's *Jogging, Aerobics and Diet* is a treatise on jogging or running combined with consideration of diet.[24]

The Ald program begins with a step test (after medical clearance) to establish your fitness and optimum level of exercise. He recommends a fifteen-week preconditioning shape-up program that involves ten minutes of warm-up and five to ten minutes of running. The Basic Time-Trainer Running Plan after the shape-up program is a twelve-week program of two phases: (1) six weeks of five-minute daily warm-ups followed by two five-minute running schedules for a fifteen-minute aerobic workout; and (2) six weeks of five-minute daily warm-ups followed by ten-minute running sets. The intermediate eighteen-week regimen requires five minutes of warm-up and twenty to thirty minutes of running. The advanced program, which lasts twelve weeks, consists of five minutes of warm-up and fifty minutes of running.

The book provides guidelines on pulse rate during exercise, with a target zone of 145—*regardless* of age. Exercises to improve flexibility and muscle strength are included.

Consumer Guide® Rating: A good jogging program with

some good training recommendations, Ald's treatise suffers its major shortcomings in prescribing a target pulse rate of 145 regardless of age and considering only one activity (jogging) for fitness training.

CURTIS MITCHELL: THE PERFECT EXERCISE

Curtis Mitchell, author of *The Joy of Jogging*, wrote another book, *The Perfect Exercise*, which advocates rope skipping for fitness.[25] Mitchell claims that jumping rope is one of the best exercises for fitness training because it is fun, easy, convenient, inexpensive, private, and open to all ages and both sexes. It strengthens the heart, reduces overweight, increases endurance, banishes flab, and improves sports skills.

Before beginning the rope-skipping program, you are to spend two weeks "getting fit to skip." Mitchell provides a series of exercises for the major joints of the body and a series of endurance tips "to accustom your feet and legs and nerves to the continuous, rhythmic overload that is necessary to develop endurance." [26] He also suggests that the workout be preceded with a warm-up and end with a cool-down period.

Two programs of rope skipping are outlined. The first, the Rodahl Program, begins with 50 skips and builds to 500 skips over a time period that is reasonable for you. The second, the Paul Smith Program, is more specific. You skip for a number of seconds or minutes, rest, skip again, etc., in a schedule of skipping "bouts." You gradually increase the skipping until you reach a total of eighteen minutes after eighteen weeks (see Figure 18). This Paul Smith Program sets target pulse rates (Figure 19).

Consumer Guide® Rating: If the Paul Smith Program is followed, *The Perfect Exercise* can be the source of a good plan. The Rodahl Program, however, is marginal; it does not

Figure 18 / The Paul Smith Rope-Skipping Program

LEVEL NO. (WEEK)	TURNS PER MINUTE	LENGTH OF EXERCISE BOUT	LENGTH OF REST PERIOD	REPETITIONS OF EXERCISE BOUT	FREQUENCY PER WEEK	TOTAL TIME OF SKIPPING DAILY
1	60	15 sec.	15 sec.	4	5	1.0 min.
2	60	15 sec.	15 sec.	6	5	1.5 min.
3	60	30 sec.	15 sec.	4	5	2 min.
4	60	30 sec.	15 sec.	6	5	3 min.
5	60	45 sec.	15 sec.	4	5	3.0 min.
6	60	45 sec.	15 sec.	6	5	4.5 min.
7	60	1.0 min.	30 sec.	6	5	6 min.
8	60	1.5 min.	30 sec.	6	5	9 min.
9	60	2.0 min.	1 min.	6	5	12.0 min.
10	60	2.5 min.	1 min.	5	5	12.5 min.
11	60	2.5 min.	1 min.	6	5	15 min.
12	60	3.0 min.	1 min.	6	5	18 min.
13	60	4 min.	1 min.	5	3–5	20 min.
14	60	6 min.	1 min.	3	3–5	18 min.
15	60	9 min.	1 min.	2	3–5	18 min.
16	60	14 min.	0 min.	1	3–5	14 min.
17	60	16 min.	0 min.	1	3–5	16 min.
18	60	18 min.	0 min.	1	3–5	18 min.

Chart from Paul Smith's book Rope Skipping: Rhythms, Routines, Rhymes, copyright © 1969, Educational Activities, Inc., Freeport, New York. Reprinted in C. Mitchell, The Perfect Exercise. NY: Simon & Schuster, 1976, p. 103

FIGURE 19 / MITCHELL TABLE OF TARGET PULSE RATES

AGE	MHRA*	FITNESS STATUS			
		SEDENTARY 65% OF MHRA	ACTIVE 75% MHRA	VERY ACTIVE 85% MHRA	RED ZONE+
20– 29	200	130	150	170	180+
30– 39	190	123	142	161	171
40– 49	180	117	135	153	162
50– 59	170	110	127	144	153
60– 69	160	104	120	136	144
over 70	150	97	112	127	135

require the number of minutes of exercise necessary to produce a training effect. The Paul Smith Program does. Furthermore, Mitchell allows for warm-up and cool-down and recommends an introductory program. Again, a short-coming here is the emphasis on a single exercise.

* MHRA = Maximum Heart Rate for Age.
+ Red Zone—Red is for danger. Until you have skipped rope for several months, you should not allow your heart to beat at a rate higher than the figure for your age shown in the Red Zone. An exercise that calls for more than 85 percent of your MHRA is for persons who are totally fit.

From C. Mitchell, *The Perfect Exercise.* NY: Simon & Schuster, 1976, p. 95.

10

REAL TOTAL FITNESS

THE CARDIOVASCULAR PROGRAMS WE HAVE LOOKED AT SO far all had the shortcoming that only one, or two at the most, of the five fitness components were emphasized. Muscle strength, muscle endurance, and flexibility were casually passed over or completely neglected. The one program that came right out and called itself *Total Fitness* had so many shortcomings that it was rated as a real washout.

Some cardiovascular programs do include specific exercises for building muscle strength and endurance and flexibility. We will take a look at some of these programs to see if we can indeed call them "total fitness" plans. The same ratings are used here as elsewhere in this book—excellent, good, marginal, poor, and not recommended. Those rated as marginal, poor, and not recommended usually fall short with respect to the amount of cardiovascular exercise they advocate.

CLAYTON R. MYERS: THE OFFICIAL "Y" PROGRAM

The Official YMCA Physical Fitness Handbook was written by Dr. Clayton R. Myers, Ph.D., Director of Physical Fitness for the National Council of YMCAs.[1]

The book begins with information on exercise physiology

and on the importance of exercise, and with advice regarding screening and testing prior to embarking on an exercise program. The program is divided into three phases—warmup, peak work, and cool-down.

Phase 1, the warm-up, lasts approximately fifteen minutes and consists of a sequence of walking and stationary exercises to prepare the body for more vigorous activity. Phase 2, peak work, lasts eighteen to twenty minutes. It consists of a series of exercises for muscle strength, muscle endurance, and flexibility, followed by cardiovascular conditioning (running/jogging/walking). During peak work, target pulse rates (80 percent of maximum) are recommended. Phase 3, the cool-down (or the warm-up in reverse) lasts five to ten minutes and is designed to return the heart rate to normal levels.

An entire session lasts forty to forty-five minutes and is repeated three times a week (See Figure 20). Myers gives specific guidelines for each phase.

In addition to this beginners' program, a "postgraduate" course of exercise is given. Here the cardiovascular training (jogging) increases from one mile up to two miles, and the muscle strength and endurance exercises are longer and more vigorous. In addition to progressive jogging, cycling, and walking programs, advice is provided for getting fit to ski.

A few problems should be noted:

1. There is room for improvement in the details of the exercise program. More time might be spent on slow stretching for flexibility. Furthermore, Myers recommends body arches, chest raises, and flutter kicks in front, all of questionable value (see Chapter 11).

2. The program may be confusing to individuals not familiar with the YMCA fitness program and its concept of continuous motion while exercising. Consequently, the charts may be misinterpreted.

FIGURE 20 / WEEKLY PROGRESSION FOR OFFICIAL YMCA BEGINNER'S EXERCISE PROGRAM

		MUSCULAR STRENGTH & ENDURANCE					CARDIOVASCULAR			
Week	Warm-up (min.)	Push-ups	Shoulder Squeezer	Flutter (sec.)	Sit-ups	Sit Tucks	Time (min.)	Jogging *	Cool-off (min.)	Total Time (min.)
1	15	6(M)	5	20	6	6	6	3 1-min. sets	10	40
2	15	8(M)	6	20	7	6	6	3 1½-min. sets	10	40
3	14	10(M)	7	20	8	10	7	3 2-min. sets	9	41
4	14	6	8	25	9	10	7	3 2½-min. sets	9	41
5	13	7	9	25	10	15	8	3 3-min. sets	8	42
6	12	7	10	30	11	15	8	3 3½-min. sets	7	43
7	12	8	10	30	12	20	9	3 4-min. sets	7	43
8	11	8	10	30	13	20	9	3 4½-min. sets	6	44
9	11	9	10	30	14	25	10	3 5-min. sets	6	44
10	10	10	10	30	15	25	10	10 min. mile	5	45

(M) is modified push-up.
* A jogging set consists of the time listed for jogging followed by two-minute recovery.

3. Dr. Neil Solomon, M.D., Ph.D., although approving the handbook as a quality program, believes that "the stress on arm and leg strength is more suited to men than women." [2] Since we think that there are no basic health reasons for differences in training programs for men and women, however, we regard Solomon's notion as a cultural bias.

4. Some people may find the program too long. But remember, the handbook outlines a program in actual use in many YMCAs across the country.

Consumer Guide® Rating: An excellent program, the YMCA plan meets the requirements for improvement of cardiovascular endurance, muscle strength, muscle endurance, and flexibility. Good information is provided on fitness and fitness testing. The handbook provides guidelines for walking, cycling, and swimming as alternatives to jogging.

THOMAS K. CURETON: PHYSICAL FITNESS AND DYNAMIC HEALTH

Physical Fitness and Dynamic Health was written by a leading figure in the cardiovascular fitness field, Dr. Thomas K. Cureton, Ph.D., now Professor Emeritus of Physical Education at the University of Illinois. The programs Cureton recommends are based on his extensive experience in over thirty years of research at the University of Illinois Laboratory, at which he conducted hundreds of workshops and fitness programs for over 600 men.

Cureton strongly believes in putting the body to use. His goal is for people to engage in an exercise program one hour a day, five to six days a week (occasionally, "in a pinch," thirty minutes is enough).

In his book *Physical Fitness and Dynamic Health*, he outlines two programs—one for home use and another for class use.[3] The typical workout in either case consists of two parts: (1) a half-hour of rhythmic warm-up of the major muscle groups to "flush the deep tissues with blood, combined with forceful breathing to gradually build up respiration" and (2) a second half-hour of running or another activity to "develop stamina and increase the efficiency of the cardiovascular system." [4]

Cureton's home-use program is divided into three phases—low gear, middle gear, and high gear. In low gear, thirty minutes are spent on ten exercises for the upper, middle, and lower third of the body. After this warm-up, thirty minutes are devoted to activities that are continuous in motion. For example:

Monday—Walk a mile or more at a good clip. Tuesday—Swim a variety of strokes, a quarter of a mile or more. Wednesday—Shovel your sidewalk or rake leaves or cut grass. Thursday—Go square dancing, or go to a gym and work out on some apparatus like a rowing machine or treadmill. Friday—Ride a bicycle three to five miles. Saturday—Play tennis, handball, or badminton. Sunday—Take an hour walk.[5]

After one month (or longer) in low gear, you move into middle gear. Again, ten exercises are to be used for a thirty-minute workout, but they are more vigorous. Instead of walking a mile, you alternate between a walk and jog for two miles. Bench stepping is also recommended.

After the middle-gear level, the high-gear program is started. The high-gear program describes ten high-gear exercises for use in the thirty-minute warm-up. This is followed by thirty minutes of endurance exercise, again upgraded: "For instance, instead of walking and jogging when you do road work, walk a mile, run a while, walk a quarter mile, sprint two hundred yards, and walk a half mile each day." [6]

For a group setting with an instructor, Cureton outlines a

series of twenty-two lessons—in low (eight sessions), middle (ten sessions), and high (five sessions) gears.

The negative aspects of the program include:

1 / The amount of time to be spent—sixty minutes, five times a week.
2 / Encouragement to sprint in middle- and high-gear programs.
3 / Recommendation of breath holding. Current research suggests that this is not a wise practice. Dr. Clayton Myers, Ph.D., for one, discourages it, especially after strenuous exercise.[7] It may cause light-headedness, a raising of blood pressure, or the valsalva phenomenon (possibly preventing blood from returning to the heart).

Consumer Guide® Rating: A fully tested and well-researched program, *Physical Fitness and Dynamic Health* may be too time-consuming or boring for some people. Cureton does not mince words or make false promises: "Don't expect a miracle. It takes a good six months to make a real improvement. And even then you can't rest on your laurels. If you do and return to your old habits, you will find that your work will have been wasted."[8]

PER-OLAF ÅSTRAND: HEALTHY AND FITNESS

Health and Fitness was written by Dr. Per-Olaf Åstrand, M.D., for the Skandia Insurance Company of Stockholm, Sweden. The booklet was then reproduced for Information Canada as part of the Canadian government's fitness thrust.[10] Dr. Åstrand, one of the world's top work physiologists, is Professor of Physiology at the College of Physical Education in Stockholm.

In his fifty-six-page booklet, Åstrand outlines a program for muscle strength and endurance, flexibility, and cardiovascular fitness. He provides training programs for home use (Program 1) and outdoors (Program 2).

In Program 1, Åstrand recommends eight to fifteen minutes of exercise using ten different exercises (Figure 21).

FIGURE 21 / ÅSTRAND PROGRAM 1

1 / Skipping or running in place for one minute, followed by a rest of ½ minute and then another work period of one minute.

2 / Sit-ups with knees bent, 16 times.

3 / Body arches, 16 times.

4 / Shoulder rolls, 24 times.

5 / Arm swings, 24 times.

6 / Arm and leg swings, 24 with each leg and arm.

7 / Hip sway, standing with feet apart, hands on hips, slowly rotating the hips.

8 / Easy skipping in place or jogging for ½ minute.

9 / Lying on the floor and extending arms with hands against the floor (strong and healthy persons) or against a sofa or chair. Do 1 to 15 push-ups with the body straight.

10 / Skipping or running in place or a step test for 1 to 5 minutes.

P.-Olaf Åstrand, *Health and Fitness.* Ottawa: Information Canada, 1975, pp. 40–43.

Program 2, for the outdoors, is the Swedish Training Track. It takes thirty to forty minutes to complete. Åstrand recommends repeating this program one or more times a week. He divides the training track program into one for the untrained and one for the trained (see Figure 22).

Åstrand also includes the following recommendations:

1 / When you're exercising, your heart rate should rise to 200 minus your age (165 for a thirty-five-year-old.)

FIGURE 22 / ÅSTRAND PROGRAM 2
PROGRAM FOR UNTRAINED OR ELDERLY PERSONS

The basic pace is ordinary walking speed. Begin leisurely and gradually increase the pace, but not so fast that you become out of breath.

5-Minute Warm-up
1 / Walking

5 Minutes of Spurt Training
2 / Take 20–30 strides at a rapid pace, preferably uphill.
3 / Recovery between spurts.

15–20 Minutes of Interval Training
4 / Brisk walk for 2–4 minute periods.
5 / Rest or slow walking between periods.
When you improve your physical condition, you can introduce intervals with jogging for 50 yards and walking for 50 yards.

PROGRAM OF PEOPLE IN GOOD PHYSICAL CONDITION

5-Minute Warm-up
1 / Alternate jogging and walking.

5 Minutes of Spurt Training
2 / Running 20–30 strides at top speed about five times, preferably uphill.
3 / Recovery between spurts.

15–20 Minutes of Interval Training
4 / Run at about 80% of top speed for 2- to 4-minute periods.
5 / Rest or jog between periods.

P.-O. Åstrand, *Health and Fitness.* Ottawa: Information Canada, 1975, pp. 44–45.

---

2 / Exercise regularly at least two or three times a week. This is to be sustained activity—brisk walking, jogging, cycling, swimming, and cross-country skiing (target pulse rate exercise).

3 / Exercise at a modest tempo; don't try to push yourself hard.

4 / Do not compete when you're out of shape.

5 / Don't exercise hard when you've had an infection.

6 / Shun laborsaving devices.

7 / Don't compete against the clock—either as a test or to get a certain number of "points" each week. (In other words, he's critical of Dr. Cooper's thirty-points-per-week approach.)

8 / In general, get at least sixty minutes of physical activity every day, not necessarily vigorous, and it doesn't have to be all at the same time.

Åstrand has little patience with the overly cautious. He raised some eyebrows with his attitude toward a medical checkup before starting training: "Everyone who is in doubt about the condition of his health should consult his physician. But as a general rule, moderate activity is less harmful for the healthy than inactivity. You could also put it this way: A medical examination is more urgent for those who plan to remain inactive than for those who intend to get into good physical shape!" [11] He is also perplexed by legal cases in which a person advised by a physician to start an exercise program suffers a heart attack and then sues the doctor. "It would be more logical for the habitually inactive person who has a heart attack to 'accuse' his physician for not warning him that inactivity was a risk factor for the development of cardiovascular disease." [12]

Shortcomings of Åstrand's program are the following:

1 / Its technical complexity. Some of the information may be beyond the understanding of the fitness novice.

2 / Most Americans will try to get by on two half-hour periods of cardiovascular exercise. *Consumer Guide®* believes that Dr. Åstrand's program would be improved if he had stressed three half-hour periods.

3 / The body arch Dr. Åstrand recommends is one of the exercises *Consumer Guide®* considers questionable (see Chapter 11).

Consumer Guide® Rating: *Health and Fitness* is rated as good. It would have been rated as excellent had Dr. Åstrand recommended exercising three days a week. The book is entertaining and offers excellent information on fitness. Åstrand presents good advice on flexibility, strength, weight control, and cardiovascular conditioning. The program is adaptable for use by people with various fitness needs. He includes specific exercises for strength and flexibility improvement.

SHEPRO AND KNUTTGEN: COMPLETE CONDITIONING

Doctors David Shepro, Ph.D., and Howard G. Knuttgen, Ph.D., both of Boston University, are respected scientists in their academic fields—Shepro in biology and Knuttgen in exercise physiology. In *Complete Conditioning: The No-Nonsense Guide to Fitness and Good Health*, they present six exercise "prescriptions": four on cardiovascular fitness, one on strength development, and one on weight control.[13]

The four on cardiovascular fitness are (1) getting started, (2) moderate intensity, (3) high intensity, and (4) super-high intensity. The "Prescription for Getting Started" is a two-month program "to get going" (see Figure 23), and calls for warm-up, easy calisthenics, walking, and running, increasing the intensity gradually.

The moderate intensity workout can be any of the three alternative activity sessions (see Figure 24), to be performed at a level of intensity that raises the heart rate to 150–160. These sessions last forty to fifty minutes.

The high-intensity workout is to be performed with the heart rate at 165–175. It, too, suggests three alternative

FIGURE 23 / SHEPRO AND KNUTTGEN:
WORKOUT FOR THE INACTIVE

SCHEDULE:

Week 1: Days 1 and 2	Warm-up; easy calisthenics 5 minutes
	Alternate jogging and walking 20 minutes
Week 1: Day 3	Warm-up; easy calisthenics 5 minutes
	Alternate jogging and walking 15 minutes
	Run at moderate pace 5 minutes
	Walk 5 minutes
Week 2: Days 1, 2, and 3	Light jogging and calisthenics 5
Week 3: Days 1, 2, and 3	minutes
	Alternate fast jog and walk 20 minutes
	Alternate moderate run and jog (as comfortable) 10 minutes
Week 4: Days 1, 2, and 3	Light jogging and calisthenics 5
Week 5: Days 1, 2, and 3	minutes
	Alternate: Moderate run 4 minutes, jog 2 minutes (repeat 4 times).
	Finish with 15-minute run at comfortable pace.
Week 6: Days 1, 2, and 3	Light jogging and calisthenics 3
Week 7: Days 1, 2, and 3	minutes
	Alternate: Moderate run 6 minutes, jog 3 minutes (repeat 3 times).
	Finish with 15-minute run (comfortable pace) but with moderate sprint for last 30 seconds of each 5-minute segment
Week 8: Days 1, 2, and 3 3 medium workouts—mix as desired.	See workouts listed for Moderate Intensity

D. Shepro and H. G. Knuttgen, *Complete Conditioning: The No-Nonsense Guide to Fitness and Good Health.* Reading, MA: Addison-Wesley, 1975, p. 57.

FIGURE 24 / SHEPRO AND KNUTTGEN
MODERATE INTENSITY WORKOUT

PURPOSE: TO BRING ABOUT MODEST
IMPROVEMENT IN CV [CARDIOVASCULAR] FITNESS.
1 / A good program for persons with modest expectations.
2 / A good beginning program for previously sedentary persons after Getting Started.

SUGGESTIONS:
1 / Don't forget the physical examination as the first step.
2 / Start slowly for the first weeks and build up the intensity slowly (or see Prescription for Getting Started).
3 / Train in attractive surroundings and with companions, if possible.
4 / Don't give up after a few tries! There will be some dull days.
5 / Use the Continuation Card to monitor your fidelity.

PROGRAM:
1 / Forty-five minutes of activity per session!
2 / Three sessions a week recommended (more if you care to).
3 / Optional daily schedules (which can be alternated):
    a. Five minutes warm-up activity; three 10-minute activity periods (heart rate, 150–160) separated by 3-minute recovery periods (jogging or walking).
    b. Five minutes warm-up activity; 5 minutes activity; 3 minutes recovery, 7 minutes activity, 3 minutes recovery, 9 minutes activity, 3 minutes recovery, 11 minutes activity (activity heart rate, 150–160).
    c. Five minutes warm-up activity; extended moderate activity for 40 minutes (heart rate of 150–160).

How to assess your progress: Take heart rate immediately after covering a set distance at a set pace, i.e., in a set time. A lower heart rate = improved CV fitness.

Typical activities are running, swimming, rowing, cross-country skiing, and bicycling. (Recovery performed at lower intensity of the same activity.)

D. Shepro and K. G. Knuttgen, *Complete Conditioning: The No-Nonsense Guide to Fitness and Good Health.* Reading, MA: Addison-Wesley, 1975, p. 54.

schedules, including higher-intensity activities and lasting forty to fifty minutes.

The three alternative schedules in the super-high-intensity workout are to be performed at 180 or higher heart rate and last about fifty minutes.

The strength-development and body-weight programs are easy to follow, comprehensive, and well planned (Figures 25 and 26).

FIGURE 25 / SHEPRO AND KNUTTGEN
STRENGTH DEVELOPMENT PROGRAM

1 / Select the body parts or movements you wish to work on and select exercise (illustrated throughout chapter) appropriate to these specific objectives.

2 / Use a resistance (generally "weights") that limits you to three to ten repetitions before fatigue, and call that a "set."

3 / With appropriate rest intervals (your preference) spacing them, perform three sets with a particular muscle group and move on to the next exercise for another group.

4 / Repeat the procedure for each muscle group and, if time permits, repeat the whole routine.

5 / Train three times each week with a similar workout each time. . . .

TO DEVELOP ADDITIONAL EXERCISES:

1 / Perform the particular movement you want strengthened.

2 / Determine what sort of activities place maximal stress on this movement.

3 / Employ those activities that best lend themselves to formal exercise and plug them into the total program.

D. Shepro and H. G. Knuttgen, *Complete Conditioning: The No-Nonsense Guide to Fitness and Good Health.* Reading, MA: Addison-Wesley, 1975, p. 64.

FIGURE 26 / SHEPRO AND KNUTTGEN
BODY WEIGHT CONTROL PROGRAM

1 / Follow your prescribed diet.
2 / Exercise at least 45 minutes a session, with 3 sessions a week as a minimum.
3 / Within each time schedule, remember that the greater the distance covered for the designated time the greater the number of calories utilized.
4 / Examples:
   a. Five minutes warm-up activity; 10 minutes of moderate-to-heavy exercise and 3 minutes moderate-to-light exercise (and repeat 2 more times).
   b. Five minutes warm-up activity; 15 minutes moderate to heavy and 5 minutes of moderate to light exercise (and repeat once again).
   c. Five minutes warm-up activity; 40 minutes of continuous moderate-to-heavy activity.
Moderate-to-heavy exercise = activity heart rate of 150–170.
Moderate-to-light exercise = activity heart rate of 125–150.

D. Shepro and H. G. Knuttgen, *Complete Conditioning: The No-Nonsense Guide to Fitness and Good Health.* Reading, MA: Addison-Wesley, 1975, pp. 65–66.

Consumer Guide® Rating: Excellent. The major shortcomings are (1) a lack of emphasis on flexibility and (2) a failure to adjust the target heart rate for age.

KIELL AND FRELINGHUYSEN: KEEP YOUR HEART RUNNING

In *Keep Your Heart Running*, Paul J. Kiell, M.D., a psychiatrist, and Joseph S. Frelinghuysen, a writer, draw a distinction between "recreational exercise" and "true fitness exercise." [14] According to these authors, games and sports are fine for recreation, but true fitness exercise consists of cardiopulmonary (aerobic) exercises—walking, running, swimming, and biking. They should be supplemented by calisthenics and weight-training exercise to improve flexibility, muscle strength, and muscle endurance; these are called "general fitness exercises."

The program is extensive. For general fitness exercise, you choose either calisthenics or weight training. Eleven calisthenic exercises are recommended (arm flinging, knee extension and flexion, alternate knee raise, double knee raise, hands overhead swinging to the floor, back exercises, figure 8, sit-ups, half knee bends, easy pull-ups, and push-ups). These are to be done in a specified period of time—six to eight minutes the first week and fifteen to seventeen minutes after forty-two weeks. After forty-two weeks your heart rate should be around 100 to 120 for the fifteen to seventeen minutes of general fitness exercises.

If you prefer, weight training can be used in place of the calisthenics. The fourteen recommended exercises are to be completed within a "time frame" of seven to eight minutes during the first week; after forty-two weeks, it takes twenty-six to twenty-seven-and-a-half minutes. Your pulse rate after forty-two weeks should be 110 to 130 immediately after the weight-training workout.

After the general fitness exercises, you are to walk/jog, starting with six tenths of a mile. By the tenth week you will have worked your way up to one-and-a-half miles (see Figure 27). The time to be spent in this activity depends on your age.

Progress throughout the program is gradual and carefully plotted out. "At the beginning of your eleventh week, if you are coming along well with your program and feel fine, you should now start to jog. Pace out fifty yards (twenty-five yards for age forty and over) so you know what it looks like

FIGURE 27 / KIELL AND FRELINGHUYSEN WALK/JOG CHART

		TIME IN MINUTES			
Week	Distance in Miles	Under Age 30	Age 30–39	Age 40–55	Age 56 and over
1	0.6	9	10½	11	11½
2	0.7	10½	12	12½	13
3	0.8	12	13½	14	14½
4	0.9	13½	15	15½	16
5	1.0	15	16½	17	17½
6	1.1	16½	18	18½	19
7	1.2	18	19½	20	20½
8	1.3	19½	21	21½	22
9	1.4	21	22½	23	23½
10	1.5	22½	24	24½	25

P. J. Kiell and J. S. Frelinghuysen, *Keep Your Heart Running*. NY: Winchester Press, 1976, p. 120.

and jog fifty (or twenty-five) yards and walk one hundred.[15] You increase the jog portion about ten yards a week and eventually reach one-and-a-half miles (in two-and-a-half to three months). Then one-tenth of a mile a week is added until you reach two miles (in twenty-five to twenty-six minutes). Next you work on reducing the time to twenty minutes (two more months). "Properly checked by your doctor, at least annually, you can add a mile or so a month to each run. Add mileage like this for six months, if twenty-five to thirty-five years old; over thirty-six, add a mile every other month, using your judgment about not getting overtired. Run long and slow during this time." [16]

Consumer Guide® Rating: An excellent program, *Keep Your Heart Running* emphasizes cardiovascular endurance, muscle strength and endurance, and body composition. Its major shortcoming is that leg flexibility is not adequately considered, and a few low-back exercises are of questionable value. The program may be too extensive or too structured for some people, but *Consumer Guide®* likes having the alternatives of weight training or calisthenics for improving muscle strength and muscle endurance.

RECREATION CANADA: THE FIT KIT

The Fit Kit was developed by Recreation Canada for the fitness and amateur sports branch of the National Health and Welfare Department of Canada. It contains an assortment of materials including the "Canadian Home Fitness Test" (a record that describes the test you are to follow), a prescription for physical activity, fit tips, fit tip progress chart, a walk-run distance calculator, an advanced version of the Canadian Home Fitness Test, and a health and fitness booklet.[17]

The record and Canadian Home Fitness Test are the most elaborate parts of the Fit Kit, prescribing how much exercise is appropriate for various age groups, discussing the step test, and offering other useful information. But the core of the fitness program is the "Prescription for Physical Activity," consisting of five steps:

1 / Move: walk, climb, ride a bike (every day, as often as possible).
2 / Stretch and deep breathe; take a fitness break and relax (daily, as needed when tense).
3 / Push, bend, twist, swing: use your body as it was designed to be used (at least three times a week).
4 / Run, swim, cycle, ski: fifteen to twenty minutes of continuous aerobic activity, vigorous enough to increase your heart rate and make you breathe deeply (at least three times a week).
5 / Enjoy life: spend time at sports, hobbies, or outdoor activities (two-hour period at least once a week).

The Recreation Canada program was intended for all age groups from children right on up through senior citizens. *Consumer Guide*® Rating: Excellent.

KAARE RODAHL: BE FIT FOR LIFE

In *Be Fit for Life*, Kaare Rodahl, M.D., director of the Institute of Work Physiology in Oslo, Norway, provides six programs: (1) the basic program; (2) the standard program; (3) the maintenance program; (4) the advanced program for men; (5) the advanced program for women; and (6) the program for men and women over sixty-five years of age.[18]

Regardless of the program selected, Rodahl provides a series of joint mobility exercises for the major joints of the body; muscle strength exercises for the arms and shoulders, abdominals, legs, back, and hands; and a rope-skipping endurance routine (see Figure 28).

FIGURE 28 / THE RODAHL MAINTENANCE PROGRAM

---

1 / ENDURANCE

Rope Skipping

Start with a 1-minute warm-up period of jumping, using any method of jumping. Rest 30 seconds and start skipping vigorously at a fast rate from foot to foot, as when running in place. Look up and keep your body erect and the back straight. Start with 100 skips the first day. Add 10 skips each day as you go along until you eventually are able to make 500 skips without stopping. As you progress, increase the speed of skipping.

2 / MUSCLE STRENGTH

Push-ups

Men: Lying face down, hands under shoulders, palms flat on the floor, straighten arms and lift body, keeping back straight and only *palms and toes* touching the floor. Extend arms fully, then bend them quickly until chest touches floor. Repeat in rapid succession 10 times. Do not hold your breath.

Women: Lying face down, hands under shoulders, palms flat on the floor, straighten arms and lift body, keeping back straight and only *palms, knees and toes* touching the floor. Extend arms fully, then bend them quickly until chest touches floor. Repeat in rapid succession 10 times. Do not hold your breath.

Knee Bends

In standing position, feet 5 inches apart, raise arms forward to shoulder height, raise yourself on toes, then bend knees slowly as far as you can, simultaneously dropping hands until fingers touch floor. Hold for 3 seconds, then straighten your knees fully again while bringing the arms up to shoulder height. Repeat 10 times.

Half V-sit

From a lying position on your back, arms at your sides, raise the legs and upper part of your body simultaneously, while at the same time you slide your hands along the thighs until the fingers touch your knees. Return to the starting position. Do this 10 times in rapid succession.

---

3 / JOINT MOBILITY

Shoulder Roll

Stand with feet apart, arms hanging loosely at your sides. Rotate the shoulders by lifting shoulder blades as in a shrug, in a circular motion. Rotate forward 10 times, then backward 10 times.

Neck Bending

Standing erect, bend your head slowly as far back as you can, then as far forward as it will go, then sideways to the left and to the right, trying to touch the shoulder with the ear. Repeat 5 times.

Kaare Rodahl, *Be Fit for Life*. NY: Harper & Row, 1966, Appendix 3.

The basic program requires five to ten minutes daily, five days a week, for three weeks. If you meet certain fitness requirements at the end of three weeks, you progress to the standard program, which takes about ten minutes, also to be done five days a week for three weeks. Again, if you meet certain fitness requirements you are then permitted to progress to the maintenance programs. These take a little less than ten minutes to complete and are to be engaged in five days a week. Those who wish and have the time to excel beyond the ordinary level of physical fitness, according to Rodahl, may progress to advanced levels, which require fifteen minutes of exercise, five days a week.

Consumer Guide® Rating: The Rodahl program is rated marginal. The book has excellent guidelines regarding fitness—especially the joint mobility program to improve flexibility and the muscle strength program for selected muscle groups. The major shortcomings are two, and the first is quite significant. Rodahl does not recommend enough time for cardio-respiratory work. The five to seven minutes of cardiovascular exercise, even though it is to be repeated five days a week, doesn't meet our minimum of fifteen to thirty minutes. Furthermore, two controversial exercises are recommended—the deep knee bend and body arches (see Chapter 11). Finally, there is no real need for a distinction between men's and women's programs.

ROSE AND MARTIN: THE LAZY MAN'S GUIDE TO PHYSICAL FITNESS

Dr. Kenneth D. Rose, M.D., former chairman of the American Medical Association's committee on exercise and physical fitness, and Jack Dies Martin, a seasoned journalist and science writer, set out to design an exercise program for the busy person. The title—*The Lazy Man's Guide to Physical Fitness*—was chosen more for its value as an eye-catcher than anything else. This book is for the person "without access to exercise areas such as parks and swimming pools, and anyone else who wants to get into better shape as simply as possible." [19]

The program claims to stress cardio-pulmonary (heart-lung) capacity and efficiency, muscle strength and muscle endurance, and flexibility exercises. To develop muscle strength, endurance, and flexibility, seven calisthenic exercises are provided, including a form of bar dips, chin-ups, bent-knee sit-ups, push-ups, walking, trunk twisters, and trunk benders. These are to be done daily, and in most instances ten repetitions of the exercise are recommended.

To achieve cardiovascular fitness, the authors suggest at

least ten minutes of strenuous exercise daily. This must be exercise that will make you breathe hard—running, jogging, running in place, walking fast, or skipping rope. Your pulse rate is to reach 70 percent of your maximum. (A week of preliminary exercising precedes this cardiovascular regimen; walk at least two miles every day in the morning or evening and do a dozen or so "jumping jacks.")

You do the calisthenics and pulse-rated exercise *daily* for four weeks; after this initial period, you are to engage in the exercises at least twice a week. Rose and Martin recommend twice a week because in their view deconditioning sets in after three days. If you are careful not to allow a nonexercise period to last more than three days, you will remain within what they call the "circle of conditioning."

Consumer Guide® Rating: The Rose and Martin approach constitutes a marginal program. The 70-percent maximum heart rate is sound, but ten minutes twice a week is not sufficient—even for maintenance of fitness. Dr. John Boyer, M.D., contends that "the half-life of exercise is about two-and-a-half days. In other words, of whatever occurs in an exercise bout, half has to be replaced every two-and-a-half days ... or three times a week." [20] Granted, this book is addressed to the busy man and woman, but the facts of fitness are the same for them as for anyone else. Extending the cardiovascular exercise segment five to ten more minutes and requesting one more day of exercise a week would be necessary to make this program adequate. Moreover, not enough attention is paid to flexibility.

BUSTER CRABBE: ENERGISTICS

Energistics was written by Buster Crabbe, former Olympic swimmer and the Tarzan, Flash Gordon, Buck Rogers, Billy Carson, and Captain Gallant of movie and television fame.

Energistics focuses on calisthenics but ties in some cardiovascular concepts.[21] Crabbe states that a fitness program should include three basic elements: a warm-up session, a period of peak exertion, and a cooling-down session. He also recommends that a good fitness program should include work on flexibility, strength, and endurance (presumably circulo-respiratory endurance). He recommends exercising a minimum of two or three times a week for twenty minutes at a target heart rate of 80 percent of maximum.

The *Energistics* program includes thirty-two exercises that work on the major areas of the body. The first six are to serve as a warm-up and a selection of the remaining twenty-six as conditioning exercises. Crabbe advises how many times a week you should engage in the vigorous exercise based on your age, health, sex, and body weight. He also gives some recommendations on exercise for starting the day, for relaxing, and on swimming.

Consumer Guide® Rating: This is a poor program. *Energistics* has some good advice on fitness but unfortunately doesn't seem to hold together:

1 / Crabbe does not recommend enough cardiovascular exercises (he suggests jogging in place twenty times). *Consumer Guide*® doubts whether the other exercises recommended and the number of repetitions will elicit proper target heart rates, except in the extremely unfit.

2 / Some of the plans at the back of the book fall short in the frequencies recommended. Three times a week should be the minimum.

3 / Some of the exercises are controversial and downright dangerous. For example, the deep knee bends, duck waddle, and body arches are potentially dangerous; and the sit-ups and leg raises as described are questionable. (See Chapter 11 for discussion of questionable exercises.)

4 / Crabbe's use of isometrics for older people is not advisable.

11

CALISTHENICS: EXERCISE BY THE NUMBERS

CALISTHENICS HAVE BEEN AROUND FOR A LONG TIME—SO long, they are an American institution. Most fitness programs, physical education classes, and athletics training plans of the 1930s, '40s, '50s, and '60s emphasized calisthenics.

Cardiovascular exercise has begun to take away some of calisthenics' thunder. In books and in fitness classes, many fitness experts are swinging away from regimens based on counting sit-ups, toe touches, and knee bends. Exercising by the numbers has seen better days.

A number of specific exercises usually included in calisthenics workouts have come under heavy fire in recent years, and we'll take a look at these individually before evaluating calisthenics programs.

CONTROVERSIAL EXERCISES

It has been charged that "at least 90 percent of the exercise programs include exercises as detrimental as they are valuable." [1] Almost any exercise can be harmful if done incorrectly, but toe touches, leg lifts, deep knee bends, body

175

arches (hyperextension of the back), toe raises, and straight-leg sit-ups have most frequently been condemned.

TOE TOUCHES

Toe touching does not trim the waistline. Dr. Allan J. Ryan, M.D., editor-in-chief of *Postgraduate Medicine* and *The Physician and Sportsmedicine,* has long advocated abolishing this exercise. "This is not an abdominal exercise, as is often explained, because the movement is accomplished by gravity, momentum, and eccentric contraction of the back extensors. The position forces the knees to overextend and places tremendous amounts of pressure on the lumbar vertebrae, a factor believed by many to have an effect on low-back complaints." [2]

Dr. W. H. Fahrni, M.D., assistant in Orthopedics, University of British Columbia Medical Faculty, believes that the repetitive touching of the toes can have a detrimental effect on the discs of the vertebral column.[3]

Doctors Philip J. Rasch, Ph.D., and Fred Allman, M.D., believe that many of the back troubles reported by housewives are caused by frequent overstretch of the spinal extensors, "resulting from their assumption of a modified toe-touch stance while making beds, dusting, picking up objects from the floor, etc. If a bouncing movement must be added to the exercise in order to touch the fingers to the toes, the insult to the joints of the lumbar spine is compounded." [4]

STRAIGHT-LEG SIT-UP

The straight-leg sit-up is often done to "strengthen the abdominals." It is not as effective as it might be because of the action of the iliopsoas muscle, one of the strongest muscles of the body. The iliopsoas, running from spinal column to femur (thigh bone), is hidden and does not give shape to the abdomen. Because of its strength, it is the muscle most likely to be used when a person sits up with legs extended. Furthermore, there is a tug on the spinal column when you sit up from this position which can cause a hyperextension of the back which can aggravate the low back. The problem is compounded if you have weak abdominal muscles.[5]

LEG LIFTS

Leg lifts done while lying on one's back have been discouraged because they can increase the severity of a particular low back ailment called lordosis. Although leg lifts were often recommended in the past as a waistline trimmer, most fitness experts (Dr. Allan Ryan, for one) have placed restrictions on this exercise or eliminated it completely.

The objections to leg lifts are basically the same as those for the sit-ups: the lifting is largely accomplished by the iliopsoas.[6]

DEEP KNEE BENDS

The forceful deep squatting of deep knee bends stretches the lateral ligaments of the knee. If the stretching is excessive, the natural protection of the knee is all but eliminated. In some instances, the cartilage of the knee can be pinched by the deep squatting.

Deep knee bends and duck walk activities have almost universally been condemned by exercise physiologists.[7] Karl Klein, of the University of Texas, a leading critic, contends that once the ligaments are stretched the knee loses its first line of defense and is predisposed to injury, particularly when struck from the side.[8]

Not all knee bends are dangerous. "Full knee bends" or "deep knee bends" refer to those in which the buttocks touch the heels of the feet. Doctors Rasch and Allman clearly state, "the safest procedure would seem to be to squat only to the point that the thighs are parallel with the floor and to eliminate completely the duck waddle and all bouncing squat movements from any exercise regimen." [9]

HYPEREXTENSION OF THE BACK

Exercises that feature hyperextension (extreme arching) of the back, either forward or backward, have been discouraged. Dr. Allan Ryan, M.D., explains, "For the large number of individuals who have varying degrees of swayback with weakened abdominals, movements which overextend the back will only exaggerate the condition and at the same time place unnecessary strain on the overused lumbar joints. . . . If subjected to repeated periods of stretching [the anterior longitudinal ligament of the vertebrae], will become permanently lengthened, consequently weakening the joint structure." [10]

In many people, weakened abdominal muscles have caused rotation of the pelvis. As a result, a hyperextension of the back occurs, and the low back muscles become stronger than the abdominals. Any body arching increases the differential between the low back and the abdominals, thereby increasing the forward curve of the spine. It is best in the beginning of any fitness program to emphasize abdominal work rather than low-back work. After the abdominals are as strong as the low-back muscles, low-back exercise can begin.

STANDING ON TOES

Allan Ryan asserts, "This exercise is questionable if it is advocated for strengthening the longitudinal arch. The exercise . . . stretches the plantar structures of the feet, which will weaken the arch." [11]

Replace this exercise with heel cord stretches or walking on the heels rather than the toes.

CORRECTING THREE MISCONCEPTIONS

CALISTHENICS DO NOT HELP YOUR HEART

In traditional calisthenics, you may begin with push-ups, which burn six to seven calories a minute and get your heart rate up to 120, and then rest a minute. You then follow with sit-ups, which may burn four to five calories a minute and increase the heart rate to 110, and rest again. The rest is the problem. There is no sustained movement. To stimulate the cardiovascular system, you must get your metabolism up and keep it up.

Unfortunately, most of the programs described in this chapter follow this alternating stop-start pattern. As a result, you get very little stimulation of the cardiovascular system or burning of calories. Calisthenics *can*, however, be effectively used for fitness training. The exercises must be put into a continuous sequence. Here is an example from one fitness book:

> Start by walking in place. Your metabolism increases, and after one minute it's up to three calories a minute. Immediately sit on the floor, perform your sit-ups, and during the entire exercise you are burning four calories. As soon as the exercise is over get up and walk in place; again your metabolism stays between three and four calories a minute. Then move into push-ups, and about thirty seconds into the exercise you're burning six to seven calories a minute. After the push-ups get up immediately and walk in place for one minute. At the conclusion of the walking move into jumping jacks.[12]

The purpose is *not* to rest between exercises. Move quickly from one to the next, with walking or running in place the only "rest" permitted.

CALISTHENICS ARE HELPFUL IN "SPOT REDUCING"

Many people assume that calisthenics will remove fat from a selected part of the body. Stationary exercises are fine for firming up specific areas where the musculature is weak. For example, if the abdomen protrudes because the abdominal muscles are weak, bent knee sit-ups, curl-ups, and V-seats will strengthen these muscles and flatten the abdomen. But sit-ups, V-seats, and curl-ups will not remove fat. To get to the bulges caused by fat deposits, you must participate in a large-muscle activity such as walking, cycling, swimming, or jogging. In other words, as one fitness writer explains, the term "spot reducing" is really a phony concept:

> Vigorous movement of a group of muscles—the arm muscles, for instance—cannot reduce or decrease the number of fat cells that lie immediately around those muscles because there is no physiological pathway for such a direct outlet. Instead, when you exercise, the nervous system triggers the release of small quantities of fat from cells all over the body. The circulatory system then picks up the fat and it is converted into energy which is used by the muscles.[13]

MUSCULAR FITNESS VERSUS CARDIOVASCULAR FITNESS

Most authors of calisthenics/circulatory exercise programs assume that people will make similar progress with respect to muscular fitness and cardiovascular fitness. That is, you will improve in both component at the same rate. Although most programs in this chapter make this assumption, it is not correct. Many times people will find that they will improve faster in cardiovascular fitness than muscular fitness or vice versa. Consequently, care must be taken when following these programs. If you find you can progress faster in muscular fitness, for example, then go to a higher level for muscular development and stay on the lower level for cardiovascular fitness development.

Considering these shortcomings, what are the advantages of calisthenic-type exercise? *The Physical Fitness Encyclopedia* acknowledges five:

1 / Calisthenics are relatively easy to learn and to perform.
2 / Very little equipment and a minimum of space are required.
3 / Vigorous workouts can be established in a short period of time.
4 / Almost all muscles or muscle groups can be developed.
5 / Free exercises can be performed alone or with a group.[14]

In addition, calisthenics do allow you to work on a particular area of your body to correct special problems or develop selected areas.

CALISTHENICS PROGRAMS

THE ROYAL CANADIAN AIR FORCE 5BX AND XBX PROGRAMS

The 5BX Program was created to provide a basis for the physical fitness of men in the Royal Canadian Air Force.[15]

The program is designed to require no equipment and a minimum amount of time (eleven minutes). It consists of six charts of five exercises each. The exercises are always performed in the same order and within the same maximum time limit. As you progress from chart to chart, slight changes in each basic exercise gradually demand more effort.

Figure 29 presents a sample chart showing the number of repetitions for the five basic exercises and the progression from the D⁻ level to the A⁺ level. Column 1 represents Exercise #1, the toe touch; #2, sit-ups; #3, body arches; #4, push-ups; and #5, running in place.

The allotted time for each exercise is noted at the bottom of each exercise. In the preliminary stages the repetitions are so few that it is fairly easy to complete the exercise routine in eleven minutes. However, as you progress upward, the activity becomes more and more demanding.

FIGURE 29 / PHYSICAL CAPACITY RATING SCALE

Level	Exercise					1-mile Run	2-mile Run
	1	2	3	4	5	In minutes	
A+	30	32	47	24	550	8	25
A	30	31	45	22	540	8	25
A−	30	30	43	21	525	8	25
B+	28	28	41	20	510	8¼	26
B	28	27	39	19	500	8¼	26
B−	28	26	37	18	490	8¼	26
C+	26	25	35	17	480	8½	27
C	26	24	34	17	465	8½	27
C−	26	23	33	16	450	8½	27
D+	24	22	31	15	430	8¾	28
D	24	21	30	15	415	8¾	28
D−	24	20	29	15	400	8¾	29
Minutes for each exercise	2	1	1	1	6		

Royal Canadian Air Force Exercise Plans for Physical Fitness. NY: Pocket Books, 1975, p. 127.

The authors recommend that you start at the very lowest level—regardless of your fitness level—and progress upward. Each person is told to progress at an age-adjusted score rate. If you are under twenty, you spend at least one day at each level; twenty to twenty-nine, two days at each level; etc., up to sixty and over, when you should spend at least ten days at each level.

The XBX program is designed to help women develop and maintain physical fitness. The writers claim it will improve general physical condition by increasing muscle tone, muscle strength, muscle endurance, flexibility and efficiency of your heart. A session takes twelve minutes, and the plan allows the exerciser to progress at her own rate. The XBX Program consists of four charts of ten exercises each. As in the 5BX Program, the charts become increasingly difficult. The ten exercises are always performed in the same order and within the same time limit (twelve minutes).

Figure 30 presents a sample XBX chart. Exercise #1 refers to toe touching; #2, knee raising; #3, lateral bending; #4, arm circles; #5, rocking sit-ups; #6, chest and leg raising; #7, side leg raising; #8, knee push-ups; #9, leg-overs; and #10, run and side jumping. The other two exercises are optional, varying from one chart to another. You begin at Level 1, moving to the next level when you can do the first without strain in twelve minutes. Continue through the levels and charts in this way until you reach the level recommended for your age group or until you feel you are exercising at your maximum capacity.

Frank Vitale, Associate Supervisor of Physical Education at the University of California at San Diego, lists five advantages of the RCAF approach: "(1) It requires no other person to assist; (2) No special equipment is needed; (3) Only a small amount of time is needed; (4) It provides a maintenance program when the desired fitness level is reached; (5) It allows for retrogression to previous levels if workouts have been missed." [16]

FIGURE 30

		1	2	3	4	5	6	7	8	9	10	8A	8B
L	24	15	16	12	30	35	38	50	28	20	210	40	36
	23	15	16	12	30	33	36	48	26	18	200	38	34
E	22	15	16	12	30	31	34	46	24	18	200	36	32
	21	13	14	11	26	29	32	44	23	16	190	33	29
V	20	13	14	11	26	27	31	42	21	16	175	31	27
	19	13	14	11	26	24	29	40	20	14	160	28	24
	18	12	12	9	20	22	27	38	18	14	150	25	22
E	17	12	12	9	20	19	24	36	16	12	150	22	20
	16	12	12	9	20	16	21	34	14	10	140	19	19
L	15	10	10	7	18	14	18	32	12	10	130	17	15
	14	10	10	7	18	11	15	30	10	,8	120	14	13
	13	10	10	7	18	9	12	28	8	8	120	12	12
Minutes for each Exercise			2		2	1	1	2	1	3	1	1	

Recommended number of days at each level ☐

Royal Canadian Air Force Exercise Plans for Physical Fitness. NY: Pocket Books, 1975, p. 30.

CRITICISMS. *Consumer Guide®* summarizes eight arguments against the RCAF plans.

1 / The programs (the 5BX especially) do not require proper warm-up, neither joint readiness nor car-

diovascular, even though the beginning exercises are quite vigorous on some charts (especially considering the time limit). *Consumer Guide*® recommends five to ten minutes' warm-up before any exercise program, whereas in these programs the entire session is eleven or twelve minutes in length.

2 / Several of the exercises recommended are questionable, e.g., sit-ups with legs straight, body arches, toes touches, and deep squats.

3 / Running in place is a good cardiovascular exercise, but it is placed at the end with no cool-down. It would have been far better to intersperse running in place between exercises, thereby providing for continuous motion.

4 / The eleven- and twelve-minute sessions do not meet our minimum requirements for cardiovascular training (fifteen to thirty minutes).

5 / Frank Vitale considers the programs "ultraconservative in establishing the starting level," and he is afraid the participant may get bored quickly before the program has a chance to provide satisfaction.[17]

6 / The programs do not allow for varying rates of progression among the different exercises. Arm and shoulder strength may progress at a faster rate than leg endurance, or vice versa, for example.

7 / On the 5BX Program, the walking and running routine at the end of Charts 1 through 5 and running routines on Charts 5 and 6 would provide the greatest cardiovascular benefit, yet receive no special notice.

8 / The programs do not allow for different rates of improvement with respect to cardiovascular fitness and muscular fitness.

Consumer Guide® Rating: 5BX and XBX are marginal programs at best.

ADULT PHYSICAL FITNESS PROGRAM—
UNITED STATES GOVERNMENT

The booklet *Adult Physical Fitness* was developed by the President's Council on Physical Fitness and Sports in an attempt to encourage the American population to get back into shape at home. It contains facts about physical fitness, a program for women, a program for men, and a discussion of how to broaden your program.[18]

Each program consists of an orientation period, a step test, and the actual exercise program. The purpose of the orientation program of mild exercise (lasting at least one and possibly two or three weeks) is to reduce the incidence of aches and pains and prepare for the more vigorous exercise. The step test is then taken, to be repeated every two weeks to see how you are improving.

The training program consists of three types of exercise: warm-up, conditioning, and circulatory. The warm-up exercises are to limber up the body and prepare the circulatory system for increased activity. Next come the conditioning exercises, designed to tone up the major muscles in the abdomen, back, and legs. The circulatory exercises stimulate the circulatory and respiratory systems (walking, running, jogging, or rope skipping).

The Council recommends that you exercise at least five days a week. There are five levels of charts, the first the easiest and the fifth the most difficult. You are to spend at least three weeks on each level. The Council expects it will take you about fifteen minutes to complete a session.

The strengths of the President's Council program are its attention to circulatory fitness, muscle strength and endurance, and flexibility. It requires little or no equipment, and the adequate warm-up is a plus.

Criticisms: Some of the criticisms lodged against the

RCAF programs can be applied as well to the President's Council plans. Several controversial exercises are recommended; the program tends to be ultraconservative in the beginning stages; and there is no cool-down.

Another drawback is the fact that the sessions last only fifteen minutes, thereby just reaching the minimum set forth by *Consumer Guide®*. Our fifteen-minute minimum refers to cardio-respiratory exercise, with warm-up time *in addition* to the fifteen minutes. In the Council program only ten minutes are spent in vigorous activity. Only at the last level for men is enough jogging recommended.

Some of the alternatives offered among the circulatory activities are not comparable. For example, on Level 2 for men, you are to pick one of the following: jog-walk for one mile, rope skip (skip one minute, rest one minute) three times, or run in place for three minutes. A jog-walk of one mile would actually be comparable to a series of eight to ten minutes of rope skipping or running in place for eight to ten minutes.

Consumer Guide® Rating: *Adult Physical Fitness* can be a good program for men and women, but only if the jog-walk sequence is followed. If the rope skipping or running in place exercises are used, this program must be rated as no better than marginal.

METROPOLITAN LIFE'S EXERCISE GUIDE

Metropolitan Life's Exercise Program for Men and Women is a modification of Level 1 of the President's Council on Physical Fitness and Sports Program.[19]

Consumer Guide® Rating: A poor program, the Metropolitan Life plan suffers the same weaknesses as the President's Council Program, and is even more drastically limited by presenting only one level.

BONNIE PRUDDEN: HOW TO KEEP SLENDER AND FIT AFTER THIRTY

Bonnie Prudden's *How to Keep Slender and Fit After Thirty* has sold extremely well over the fifteen years since it was first published.

According to Prudden, the ideal exercise schedule includes five minutes of warm-up, fifteen minutes of exercise for specific areas, thirty minutes of sports (running and jumping, floor progressions, mat work, apparatus, weights), five minutes of cooling off, and, if time permits, five minutes of relaxation (Figure 31).[20] She does not insist on this time allotment, however, and leaves the total time up to the exerciser. You can omit any segment of the program except the warm-up.

Prudden's warm-up consists of thirteen exercises working the major muscle groups and joints. She then provides a whole series of exercises for problem areas—e.g., hips, thighs, abdominals, feet—and general fitness.

Bonnie Prudden's book has some strong points that deserve special attention. She includes excellent advice on taking stock of yourself—past, present, and future. *Consumer Guide*® believes that exercise books should all provide such a good starting basis to keep you from floundering. The book's guidance on establishing a workout routine (Figure 31) is clear and flexible, allowing for individual variation yet setting good minimal requirements. Another strong point is the firm insistence on adequate warm-up. And, finally, *How to Keep Slender and Fit After Thirty* describes some excellent exercises for conditioning major muscle groups of the body.

CRITICISMS: Prudden recommends massage for removing fatty deposits. In Chapter 18 we will explain that your body just doesn't work that way and that the concept of massage as a fat-remover is erroneous. Prudden implies throughout

FIGURE 31 / BONNIE PRUDDEN'S EXERCISE SCHEDULE

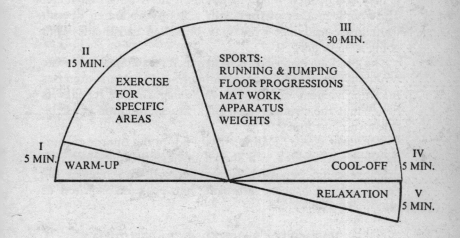

III
30 MIN.

II
15 MIN.

SPORTS:
RUNNING & JUMPING
FLOOR PROGRESSIONS
MAT WORK
APPARATUS
WEIGHTS

EXERCISE
FOR
SPECIFIC
AREAS

I
5 MIN.

WARM-UP

COOL-OFF

IV
5 MIN.

RELAXATION

V
5 MIN.

Bonnie Prudden, *How To Keep Slender And Fit After Thirty*. NY: Pocket Books, 1970. p. 71.

the text that spot reducing works. We've made it clear in this chapter that spot reducing does not work.

How to Keep Slender and Fit After Thirty emphasizes muscle fitness rather than cardiovascular fitness. Bonnie Prudden would probably not agree with that statement, but it comes through loud and clear in the book. For example, she states, "Without question most (if not all) would profit from some endurance exercise, but many could never come close to the thirty points demanded by the exponent of aerobics [twenty to thirty minutes three times a week]. Even if they could, their *wants,* if not their needs, are elsewhere. The young mother of four with a floppy abdomen doesn't want to be told that what may be called calisthenics isn't going to help her." [21]

The Prudden approach is to fit specific exercises to specific problems—exercises for overcoming round sholders, exercises for improvement of sex, etc. *Consumer Guide*® repeats its belief that the primary goal of a fitness program must be cardiovascular fitness.

Consumer Guide® Rating: If you adopt the outline recommended by Prudden and shown in her schedule chart, the program must be rated as excellent. If you neglect the cardiovascular aspects, however, her program is rated as marginal.

MARJORIE CRAIG: MISS CRAIG'S 21-DAY SHAPE-UP PROGRAM FOR MEN AND WOMEN

Miss Craig's 21-Day Shape-Up Program for Men and Women was written by Marjorie Craig, a graduate of Arnold College (now Bridgeport University at Bridgeport, Connecticut) who has worked in muscular rehabilitation at the Neurological Institute of the Columbia Presbyterian Medical Center and at Richard Hudnut's. She now teaches private exercise lessons at Elizabeth Arden's in New York City and is supervisor of the salon's body department.

The 21-Day Program consists of thirty-five exercises.[22] You do twelve of them the first few days, adding new ones day by day and increasing the number of times each exercise is done. At the end of the twenty-one days, you are doing all thirty-five. A chart at the bottom of each page pinpoints daily changes in the routine.

In addition to the 21-Day Program, Craig gives exercises for specific areas, for relief of tension, and for post-pregnancy, as well as a section devoted to body movement. She pays much attention to preventing back pain and recommends movements to prevent back ailments.

The Craig book includes discussion of muscle tone, strength, and firmness, and the relationship of these factors to physical fitness. It also explains how regular exercise, at least thirty minutes a day, helps prevent degenerative diseases and slows down the physical deterioration associated with aging.

Consumer Guide® Rating: A book with excellent exercises and precautions, Miss Craig's program's major shortcoming is that it neglects specific attention to cardiovascular fitness. As a result, the program is rated marginal. Inclusion of a cardiovascular exercise routine of twenty minutes would place it in the excellent category.

SOLOMON AND HARRISON: DR. SOLOMON'S PROVEN MASTER PLAN FOR TOTAL BODY FITNESS AND MAINTENANCE

Dr. Neil Solomon, M.D., Ph.D., and Evalee Harrison wrote *Dr. Solomon's Proven Master Plan for Total Body Fitness and Maintenance* because dieters on *Dr. Solomon's Easy, No-Risk Diet* [23] complained that after losing weight they didn't like their figures. He and his sister set out to help dieters firm up.

The Master Plan outlines a series of twenty-four exercises for seven basic positions. Areas of the body to be worked on include the neck, shoulders, arms, waist, midriff, legs, feet, ankles, abdomen, spine, hips, thighs, and buttocks. The plan progresses from a warm-up phase through attainment of fitness and then into maintenance.

Solomon and Harrison include a section on extra exercise for special areas of concentration. Advice is given on family fitness, how to build fitness into your traveling, and how to be sexier.[24]

Consumer Guide® Rating: Similar to most other calisthenics programs, Dr. Solomon's comes up short on cardiovascular fitness, although the authors do recommend walking, jogging, and sports. They are not specific, however, in telling the reader how to progress. They also recommend a few of the exercises we've singled out as controversial. The book implies that spot reducing works. The program is rated as poor.

MAGGIE LETTVIN: THE BEAUTIFUL MACHINE

Maggie Lettvin's *The Beautiful Machine* consists of a sixty-four-page planning guide and 180 exercise cards designed to make your body slimmer, stronger, healthier—and a more beautiful machine.[25] On each card, Lettvin demonstrates and describes each exercise. With the help of the sixty-four-page exercise-planning guide, the exerciser selects the cards (easy, medium, and hard) best suited to his or her needs and physical condition.

Programs are provided for practically every part of the body. On abdomens, for example, she considers total sag, front, side, lower (for pot-bellies), specials for the waistline, and flexibility. It's that way with practically every major segment of the anatomy.

Lettvin provides advice and exercise for circulo-respiratory endurance, flexibility, muscle endurance, posture, and post-pregnancy. Exercises as therapy are also given—for varicose veins, whiplash, bad backs, breathing problems, hernias, and after surgery.

Consumer Guide® Rating: Similar to other calisthenics programs, *The Beautiful Machine* is rated marginal because it does include a cardio-respiratory emphasis, but no progression schedule, leaving the serious exerciser stranded.

GLENN SWENGROS: FITNESS WITH GLENN SWENGROS

Fitness with Glenn Swengros [26] was written by Glenn Swengros, former Program Director of the President's Council on Physical Fitness and Sports, and John J. Monteleone, a professional writer. It was designed to be "the first complete exercise book with something for everyone."

Swengros provides general conditioning exercises for men, women, children, and young adults. He also recommends a program for executive fitness—that is, for the busy traveling executive. Exercise programs are given for during and after pregnancy, and he provides a series of toning exercises for different areas of the body. A series of exercises is also provided for improvement of flexibility, muscle strength, and muscle endurance for various sports that you might participate in; and finally, walking and jogging programs are included.

Consumer Guide® Rating: A good book with good programs for specific problems, *Fitness with Glenn Swengros* encourages continuous motion from one exercise to another. That increases the effectiveness of the exercise as a calorie burner and for conditioning the heart and lungs. He recommends thirty minutes of exercise, three to five times a week.

12

YOGA—STRETCHING FOR FITNESS

OVER 300 BOOKS ON YOGA ARE CURRENTLY AVAILABLE, AND there are over 60 books on Hatha (physical) Yoga alone. This quantity in itself makes it necessary to select a focus. Risking the wrath of the yoga practitioners of the world, *Consumer Guide®* will consider Hatha Yoga as a general program rather than evaluating each plan separately.

Obviously, the major problem with this approach is that it overlooks differences in individual programs. *Consumer Guide®* recognizes this limitation, yet feels that this is the most logical way to proceed, considering the large number of plans available.

WHAT IS YOGA?

According to Dr. Allan Ryan, M.D., "Yoga is one of the six classic systems of Hindu philosophy. It is characterized chiefly by its emphasis on the importance of body control and achieving union (which is what the word 'yoga' means) with the object of all knowledge. In the case of those who practice yoga as a religious way of life, the object is Brahma, the universal spirit. In the case of the atheists, it becomes deeper knowledge of self." [1]

Yoga has several branches or divisions, but the goal of all is the same—union with the Supreme Consciousness. Each division is based on a particular approach to this goal. In Karma Yoga, for instance, it is achieved through work and action; in Jnana Yoga, through knowledge and study; in Bhakti Yoga, through devotion and selfless love; in Mantra Yoga, through invocations and sounds. The highest form of yoga is Raja Yoga (Royal Yoga), the yoga of consciousness.[2]

HATHA YOGA

In Hatha Yoga, union with the Supreme Consciousness is approached through a series of body attitudes (postures) and breathing exercises. The main postures (asanas) consist of stretching, head and shoulder stands, balancing, standing, and sitting postures. A yoga workout typically combines groups of these postures, the movements of getting into and out of them, relaxation, and simple breathing exercises.[3] Various asanas can be grouped so that specific body parts are exercised.

In most programs, a mastery of the various asanas and breathing techniques can be expected after about four to twelve weeks of regular (twenty to thirty minutes daily) practice. Yogis (those who practice yoga) prefer a period of solitude and a regular time of day. Some exercises may take years or more to achieve. Indeed, some postures may never be mastered (primarily because of age or orthopedic disability).

According to yogis, "The results of the practice of Hatha, or physical, yoga are equated with what are supposed to be the characteristics of youth. Richard Hittleman, the most prolific U.S. writer on the subject, notes that people who practice yoga will have improved: flexibility; grace; serenity; relaxation; sleep; vitality; endurance; circulation; strength of vital organs and glands; firmness and strength of muscles;

taut, smooth skin; weight; recovery; alertness; and clarity of mind." [4]

The art of yoga is over 5,000 years old. Modern-day health concepts may or may not have disproved the theories of the "old masters" regarding the benefits of yoga. *Consumer Guide*® regards some of the claimed benefits as central to physical fitness and feels that an evaluation of these claims in light of current research is certainly appropriate.

FLEXIBILITY

Richard Hittleman notes, and other yogis agree, that you are to "do each asana slowly and exactly as described. Do not strain. If you cannot achieve the extreme position ... don't worry. Stretch only as far as is comfortable. While you are holding that position, relax. If you feel tension in one of your muscles concentrate on relaxing it." [5] This advice on how to do yoga exercises remarkably parallels the statements made earlier about improvement of flexibility; the stretch is to be slow, sustained, and not ballistic. Dr. Herbert deVries, Ph.D., lists three distinct advantages of static exercise:

1 / There is less danger of going beyond the safe limits of stretching, since the exerciser moves into position slowly and stops before harm is done. With ballistic exercises, the exerciser may realize too late that he or she has passed the limit.

2 / The energy cost is lower for static stretching, so the exercises don't tire the athlete for other activities.

3 / Ballistic exercises may cause muscle soreness; static stretching tends to relieve muscle soreness. [6]

Dr. George A. Sheehan, M.D., reports: "Although most athletes, fans, and physicians still view such tragedies (muscle pulls, tears, and strains) as acts of God, there is a growing awareness that these injuries are not accidental, that they can even be predicted and prevented. Acting on this idea, three pro-football teams, the Steelers, the Broncos, and the Redskins, now employ 'flex' coaches to direct the players in stretching exercises." [7]

Research, logic, and experience indicate that yoga exercises are very effective in improving flexibility. Caution must be exercised, however, not to get into extreme positions without proper conditioning. Allan Ryan, in his critique of yoga, wrote, "Unsupervised attempts ... to assume some of the more difficult postures might result in some harm to the untrained individual." [8]

Consumer Guide® Rating: Many of the yoga postures provide an excellent way to improve flexibility, but the extreme postures are not necessary for the average person. Anyone on an aerobic program such as running, walking, or cycling should definitely consider including selected yoga postures or a yoga program for flexibility development.

REDUCTION OF STRESS AND TENSION

The problem in trying to evaluate yoga's contribution to relieving stress and tension is that we may be extending beyond the realm of Hatha (physical) Yoga. Other branches of yoga may be more relevant in this area, but this discussion is limited to the role of Hatha Yoga.

Doctors Wynn F. Updyke, Ph.D., and Perry B. Johnson, Ph.D., of the University of Toledo, assert that yoga can be used to reduce mental tension resulting from emotional strains: "Some moderns think of yoga as an extended system of psychotherapy; others regard it as an excellent technique to gain relief from tension." [9] Research tends to support this concept. Dr. Nicholas G. Alexiou, M.D., medical director of the Employee Health Service of the New York State Department of Civil Service, states that Shavasan (a yogic breathing exercise) can ease the tension brought on by the pressures of everyday living. He has observed that normal adults over fifty have a tendency to build up tension, possibly because people become more introspective with maturation. They explore the emotional and intellectual spheres and tend to neglect physical activity. Investigators found that the practice of Shavasan significantly reduced tension.[10]

Other studies suggest that Hatha Yoga in conjunction with other branches of yoga may be helpful in altering in a positive manner the responses of the autonomic nervous system.[11]

Consumer Guide® Rating: It has yet to be proven that yoga will help in relieving stress and tension, but this is a promising field of investigation. *Consumer Guide®* concludes that claims regarding yoga's ability to reduce tension and stress, increase sleep and serenity, etc., are not excessive. The only question is whether all this can happen through Hatha Yoga alone.

ENDURANCE

A person who is overly tense, unable to sleep, etc., will obviously have decreased vitality and endurance. A reduction of tension and stress will allow that person to *return* to normal levels. What we have been talking about in this book, however, is *improvement* of vitality and endurance—not just a return to a previous level.

Yogis have also made the claim that standard exercises are the height of folly because they waste energy. Instead they advocate "conserving" energy: "The cat is the classical example of this conservation of energy. He seems to have the ability to store energy so that it is always available to him as needed. He does no setting-up exercises, but he *does* exercise. How? Watch him carefully and you will observe that he is continually *stretching*."[12]

The yogis miss the point here. A cat does more than

stretch. It runs, jogs, walks, leaps, races, and climbs. It is an aerobic animal. This can be taken one step further. A wild cat, such as a tiger, lion, cougar, or panther, stretches but also runs, leaps, etc., and is trim, vital, and has fantastic endurance. Place this animal in a zoo and its stretching continues, but its physique goes to pot and the cat becomes lazy. Why? No aerobic work.

Relatively few studies have been conducted on yoga and endurance. Those that have shown favorable results reached their conclusions based on the study of just one subject— hardly a reliable basis for firm general conclusions.[13] Two studies concerning *groups* of subjects found that physical efficiency benefits of yoga occurred with respect to breath-holding and forced expiratory flow. No changes were noted in ventilation/minute volume, rate of respiration, oxygen consumption, pulse rate, blood pressure, mechanical efficiency, maximum breathing capacity, and maximum oxygen uptake—the real fitness measures.[14]

Dr. Allan Ryan, M.D., observed in his examination of yoga and fitness, "The few functional tests on practitioners of yoga that have been performed indicate relatively poor function, certainly below any level which would be consistent with what we define as physical fitness." [15]

Consumer Guide® Rating: Yoga does not improve endurance. Research in exercise physiology has established that to build energy you must expend it. Conserving energy will actually reduce your store. A reduction in stress and tension and improvement in relaxation may get a person back to what was normal prior to stress and tension, but it does not improve endurance per se. Improvement requires large-muscle activities of a continuous nature. Consequently, the claim that yoga improves vitality and endurance is not justified.

MAINTENANCE OF PROPER CIRCULATION

One well-known claim is that yogis are able to slow and possibly stop their heartbeat at will.[16] Doctors M. A. Wenger, B. K. Bagchi, and B. K. Anand concluded in their study that these claims were based on misinterpretations of data.[17] Dr. Allan Ryan, reviewing this research, offers an explanation:

> The control of the heart rate, which is said to be an accomplishment of the more experienced practitioners, can be established for brief periods by performing the Valsalva maneuver, attempting to exhale forcefully against a closed glottis. This may cause an apparent arrest of the heart by diminishing the peripheral pulses to the point where they cannot be detected by palpation. ... Nevertheless, an electrocardiogram taken at this time will show a regular but reduced heart rate, perhaps with an increase in the P-R interval or decrease or disappearance of the P wave.[18]

Along with the decreased heart rate, improved cardiac function is another reported benefit of yoga—that is, more blood pumped with each beat of the heart. Again, Dr. Ryan disagrees: "There is no reason to believe from a conceptual analysis of yoga practices that the ability of the heart to increase the efficiency of the circulation or to recover from strenuous exercise improves." [19] Furthermore, a study conducted by H. S. Nayar, R. M. Mathur, and R. S. Kumar showed no significant change in pulse rate.[20]

Another claim is that yoga can effect a decrease in elevated blood pressure. Here, too, the research conclusions are mixed. Nayar, Mathur, and Kumar found no change in blood pressure (the subjects had normal blood pressures).[21] On the other hand, Dr. Herbert Benson, M.D., reported a decrease in elevated blood pressure in his subjects.[22] Optimistic conclusions were also reached in work by Dr. C. H. Patel reported in *The Lancet*. Dr. Patel used yoga relaxation and biofeedback techniques in the treatment of twenty patients for hypertension. As a result of this approach, antihypertensive therapy was stopped altogether in five patients and blood pressure reduced by 33 percent to 60 percent in another seven patients. Blood pressure control was better in four others. Only four did not respond to the therapy. His conclusion was that the results confirmed a useful new approach in the treatment of hypertension.[23] Finally, Doctors K. K. Datey, S. N. Deshmukh, C. P. Dalvi, and S. L. Vinekar demonstrated that yogic exercise (proper breathing) will reduce blood pressure in hypertensive patients provided that there is complete mental and physical relaxation.[24] Interestingly, some yoga practitioners and observers caution against inverted yoga postures for people with high blood pressure, arteriosclerosis, or other heart disease.[25]

Consumer Guide® Rating: There is not enough evidence to support the contention that yoga will maintain proper circulation. *Consumer Guide*® does feel that yoga may be helpful in relieving hypertension in selected individuals. This is not a recommendation for self-treatment; the subject should be discussed with your physician.

STRENGTH OF THE VITAL ORGANS AND THE GLANDS

Some yoga practitioners claim that selected postures may help cure arthritis, the common cold, diabetes, gall bladders, menstrual disorders, piles, and many other ailments.[26] Others are more moderate and make less extravagant claims but do feel that the inverted position will stimulate the thyroid gland, help maintain good vision and hearing, help prevent hardening of the arteries, improve the complexion and the condition of the scalp and hair, and help pass kidney stones.[27]

Consumer Guide® Rating: The claims that yoga strengthens the vital organs and glands is unfounded. *Consumer Guide*® has been unable to find research to support the claims. Reputable practitioners avoid such statements, and readers should regard these claims with skepticism.

FITNESS AND STRENGTH OF THE MUSCLES

Dr. Allan Ryan's statement on yoga and muscle strength provides an adequate summary:

As a practical matter, muscle strength may be somewhat increased in certain groups due to the dynamic tension brought about in maintaining some of the postures over extended periods of time. These are not necessarily muscle groups which would be used much in work or sports activities, and, therefore, overall strength may not be increased as measured by conventional estimates of this aspect of general physical fitness. Because there is some relationship between weight and strength, and because the diet of orthodox yoga practitioners is lactovegetarian, disposing them to be lean and not well-muscled, strength seems to be below the average for persons otherwise similar as to age and height.[28]

Consumer Guide® Rating: Yoga may increase the firmness and strength of some muscles, but not enough to increase general fitness. Traditional calisthenics are far superior to yoga in this regard.

TAUT, SMOOTH SKIN

Richard Hittleman and others believe that yoga can help correct wrinkles, poor complexion, and sallow skin in the face and throughout the body. He attributes these problems to poor blood circulation and claims that the practice of yoga will lead to improved skin tone.[29]

Consumer Guide® Rating: *Consumer Guide®* has been unable to find evidence supporting the notion that taut, smooth skin is a by-product of yoga practice.

WEIGHT REGULATION

Probably the second most popular claim about yoga is that it will help you lose weight, trim inches, remove unsightly flab, and firm up muscles. To support these contentions, personal testimonials and "before and after" pictures are used.

It has been reported that Hatha Yoga uses up approximately 195 to 230 calories per hour.[30] Most yoga sessions last around half an hour, so that the average person burns a hundred or so calories per session. These same people would have used about thirty calories during that half-hour even if sleeping or watching TV, so the net is only around seventy calories a day. That would be around seven pounds a year, a small contribution to weight control. And evaluation of yoga's potential in weight control is complicated by the fact that many practitioners combine the exercise with yogic dietetic practices—a lactovegetarian diet and fasting (partial or complete). Consequently, the weight loss reported may be due to the diet and fasting rather than the activity.

Yogis assert that the real contribution of yoga to weight control or regulation comes with the inverted position. In this position, they say, the thyroid gland, which plays a critical role in weight loss or gain, is stimulated.[31]

Since there is no such thing as spot reducing, the claim that selected yoga positions will burn fat off a particular part of the body must be discounted. Certain yoga positions may, however, improve physique through muscle development.

Consumer Guide® Rating: Yoga's contribution to weight regulation is meager. The activity of yoga is better than no activity (sleeping or watching TV), but there are better approaches (discussed in Chapter 14) to weight control. The most effective are big-muscle activities such as walking, cycling, swimming, etc. Particular areas of the body may be firmed up with specific exercises so that a selected muscle becomes stronger and tauter to give the appearance of lost inches.

Consumer Guide® does feel, however, that if a person overeats because of stress and tension—and if this same person finds yoga relaxing—the practice of Hatha Yoga may help control the compulsive eating and thereby aid in weight control.

CONSUMER GUIDE® SUMMARY

1 / Yoga can improve flexibility and grace.

2 / Yoga does not improve endurance.

3 / Yoga is probably a good way to release tension and stress.

4 / Yoga does not maintain proper circulation (although it may be helpful in reducing elevated blood pressure).

5 / Yoga does not improve the strength of the vital organs and glands.

6 / Yoga may improve the firmness and strength of selected muscles and muscle groups.

7 / Yoga does not produce a taut, smooth skin.

8 / Yoga's concepts of weight control are questionable.

Thus, yoga is a good program to use for improvement of flexibility and as an adjunct to other more vigorous types of sports such as walking, cycling, swimming, tennis, etc. As an overall fitness program, however, yoga merits a poor rating.

13

MUSCLES, MANHOOD, AND THE NINETY-SEVEN-POUND WEAKLING

MANY PEOPLE PLACE GREAT VALUE ON BULGING MUSCLES. Most of us remember the ninety-seven-pound weakling who had sand kicked in his face and lost his girl friend to the beach bully. Then, after a few short weeks he came back to the beach with newly developed Charles Atlas muscles and got his revenge.

That ad campaign was years ago, yet many people still identify health, success, and masculinity with big muscles. A quick look through the current crop of men's magazines makes that clear. A survey by *Psychology Today* showed that 19 percent of their male readers and 21 percent of their female readers believed that strength was an important characteristic of masculinity.[1]

Women, too, are beginning to take an interest in developing their own strength. Nowadays more and more women are lifting weights or engaging in other strength-building exercise. Once afraid that strong muscles would be unattractive and "unfeminine," women are questioning the wisdom of self-imposed "weakness." Often for much the same reasons as men—to develop self-confidence, health, a capacity for self-defense, etc.—women enter rigorous strength-building programs. The results are fitness benefits, and no bulging biceps after all. Work done by Dr. Jack Wilmore, Ph.D., indicated that a woman "can make rapid gains in strength, reaching levels she never thought possible. ... Most important, she won't develop large muscle masses. On the contrary, the hard work of lifting weight enhances her figure." [2] The reason for this is that "the male hormone, testosterone, is responsible for muscle bulkiness in males. Testosterone is present in women, but the amount is probably too low to have any substantial effect on their muscle size." [3]

HOW STRONG DO WE NEED TO BE?

A minimum amount of strength is a prerequisite for endurance, flexibility, and skill. If you are not strong enough, jogging is virtually impossible because of low back pain. In order to cycle, you have to be strong enough to turn the pedals. So strength is a necessary training factor. Yet the amount of strength a person needs is hard to pin down.

WHAT ABOUT MUSCLE ENDURANCE?

Muscle endurance, the ability of a muscle or group of muscles to do repeated exercise or contractions, is closely related to muscular strength. You obviously need a minimal amount of strength to develop endurance. For example, if you are unable to do one modified push-up (minimum strength), you can't begin to work on endurance for that exercise, which would require repetition of fifteen to thirty.

Recent research indicates that working on either of these two components enhances the other to some degree.[4] In general, muscle strength is improved by high-resistance, low-repetition exercise, and muscle endurance is improved by low-resistance, high-repetition exercise. But some improvements in either component can be expected while working on the other (at least for the average exerciser).

STRENGTH AND ENDURANCE FOR WHAT?

At least four motivation patterns can be discerned among those who engage in strength and muscle-endurance exercise. Many people are motivated by a combination of these and other factors.

First are those who engage in strength-building exercise as an adjunct to an overall exercise program. They may want more muscle definition—enough to look attractive, but not a large muscle mass. They may want more strength, too, but the primary goal in adding such exercise is often to look better and firm up flabby muscles.

A second motivation behind strength-building exercise is to improve sports performance.

Third, others may engage in strength exercise in order to compete with other people, as in weight-lifting competition.

Last are the body builders. These are the men who lift weights to develop massive physiques for posing and display.

HOW MUSCLE STRENGTH IS DEVELOPED

Strength-building techniques fall into three categories: isometrics, isotonics, and isokinetics. Isometric exercises contract muscles without producing movement; placing your two hands in front of you and pushing them together is an example. Isotonic exercises refer to muscle contractions that require movement; calisthenics and weight training are examples. Isokinetic exercises refer to those that involve movement with controlled resistance. That is, the faster you try to move, the more resistance you meet; and the slower you move, the less resistance. Typical examples are the programs carried out with the *Apollo Exer-Gym*, and *Exer-Genie* devices.

All three techniques work. Temple University's Dr. Richard Berger, Ph.D., explains, "Muscles don't have eyes. To increase strength, you've got to use heavy resistance and there are several ways to do that. You can use barbells, cables, your own body weight, a towel, or a rope. It really doesn't matter as long as you provide enough resistance."

How much resistance? The answer is the same as before: It depends upon the individual—how much strength you have to begin with and how much you want.

ISOMETRIC PROGRAMS

Isometric exercises have received a good bit of attention over the last few years. Because they involve no body movement, it looks as though no effort is required. It is also said to be a "fast" method in that only ten seconds or so of exertion are needed to build strength of selected muscle groups.

In isometric exercise, a muscle or group of muscles is exerted against an immovable object, which may be a wall, a bar, a taut rope, a towel, or another set of muscles.

Isometrics were introduced to the public in the 1920s when Charles Atlas published his *Dynamic Tension* Course.[5] It was not until the 1960s, however, that isometrics began to receive a good deal of attention from professionals and consumers. The impetus came with the translation by the late Dr. Arthur Steinhaus, Ph.D., of the work of two German researchers, T. Hettinger and E. A. Muller, whose experiments showed that isometric exercise could produce strength gains of approximately 5 percent a week.[6] However, subsequent investigations reported that 2 percent a week was more realistic,[7] and that isometrics were helpful in building only one component of fitness (strength).

"Instant, effortless exercise" was here, and the claims were numerous and dramatic. Supposedly, waistlines could be trimmed, longevity increased, weight reduced, posture improved, facial wrinkles removed, stamina increased, strength developed, new energy found, and sports performance improved—all with no-sweat exercise of five or fewer minutes a day. Programs such as *Ten Static Exercises,* [8] *Isometric Exercises,* [9] *How to Exercise Without Moving a Muscle,* [10] *Facial Isometrics,* [11] and a host of similar books glutted the market in the 1960s. But then came reports that isometrics were not so fantastic.

CRITICISMS OF ISOMETRIC EXERCISES

As the popularity of isometrics increased, so did the research and investigation into their effectiveness as a means of achieving fitness. The past ten years' work has fairly well defined isometrics' contribution to fitness.

1. In one report, Doctors Jay A. Bender, Ph. D., Harold M. Kaplan, Ph.D., and Alex Johnson, Ph.D., state simply and clearly, "Isometric exercises are not the whole answer to the conditioning needs of most people." [12] Dr. H. Harrison Clarke, Ed.D., agrees: "Physical fitness is more than muscular [strength] or even muscular endurance. The third essential component is pulmonary-circulatory endurance. Thus, any exercise program limited solely to strength development by any method is deficient as an adequate approach to physical fitness." [13] What these experts are saying, of course, is that isometric exercise is effective only to develop strength, and that the other components of fitness are necessary. In fact, the most important component—circulo-respiratory endurance—is entirely neglected.

2. Isometric exercise may be dangerous for heart disease patients. Dr. O. A. Matthews, M.D., of the University of Texas Southwestern Medical School in Dallas, found that eleven of twenty-three patients with arteriosclerotic heart

disease developed arrhythmias during isometric exercise. Furthermore, of eighteen patients with valvular heart disease, five had arrhythmias during isometric exercise. And two of three patients with myocardial disease developed arrhythmias during isometric exercise. He also found that 78 percent of the patients developed premature ventricular contractions; 20 percent of the patients developed these during isometric exercise. He recommended that heart patients not engage in any type of isometric exercise.[14]

3. According to Dr. Jay Bender and his colleagues, isometric exercise using the whole body or larger groups of muscles may fail to achieve the desired effect. "That would include exercise programs as pressing the whole body against a bar or applying gross resistance with ropes or straps and without the benefit of measurement. Such programs may develop the wrong muscles, partly through unwanted muscular substitution and partly because of failure to use the full range of motion about the joints." [15]

4. Neglect of flexibility is quite a problem with isometrics. While the exercises improve strength, they may be causing a decrease in flexibility. If forced to trade off one fitness component for another, *Consumer Guide*® would emphasize flexibility over muscle strength. Closely allied with this is the observation that isometrics may increase the vulnerability to joint damage.[16]

5. In isometrics it is difficult to know if you are exerting enough to make an improvement. For one thing, isometric exercises are very specific. You exercise one muscle area at a time. One writer explains that "if you are interested in general conditioning, it is as time consuming as anything else. Because isometrics are so specific you have to work all parts of the body to make sure you are getting at the whole area." [17] It's also difficult to know how much exertion to put into each exercise. Hettinger and Muller had found that to make 5-percent gains in strength you had to contract at two thirds of your maximum for six seconds.[18] But you have no

way of knowing whether you are exerting 20 percent, 50 percent, or 100 percent.

6. Lack of motivation is another reported problem. It's hard to say whether this is because people attracted to isometrics were not really interested in exercise to begin with (that's why they chose a type in which you don't even have to move) or because the activity itself is boring. Hal Higdon reported that Dr. W. D. Paul, M.D., team physician for the University of Iowa, found that football players could concentrate on only one or two isometric exercises. "If they have a great number of exercises to do, they'll start cutting them down as fast as possible." [19] Other authorities have reported this problem as well.

7. The benefits of isometric exercise are often overrated. Phrases such as "no-sweat exercise," "effortless exercise," "exercise only three minutes a day," and "how to remove inches without moving a muscle" are common in advertising. The same ads report that successful individuals, athletic teams, beauty queens, and movie stars trim down and get into shape with this new miracle form of exercise. Almost all the claims stressed in advertising about isometric exercise are false and misleading.

REBUTTALS

1. Whether the 2-percent- or 5-percent-a-week figure is correct, isometric exercise is an effective way to increase strength. Research shows that strength and muscle size do increase, and muscle definition and appearance therefore will improve.

2. Isometric exercises may be of great therapeutic value. For example, for a person with a knee in a cast, isometric exercise can help prevent the thigh muscle from atrophying excessively. This is true of any area where a joint cannot be moved.[20]

3. Isometric exercises can be done practically anywhere—

shopping, sitting in an office, automobile, watching television, etc. They are simple and effective.

4. Little time or equipment is needed. As a result, isometrics have been recommended as the most efficient way to gain muscle strength.

5. Isometric exercises are effective in reducing the waistline—*if* lack of strength of abdominal muscles is the cause of sagging abdomen.

6. Isometrics can be used to develop strength for a particular movement. *The Physical Fitness Encyclopedia* explains, "A golfer can position his body and club in such a manner that will simulate contact with the ball. By exerting his body maximally in that position, the muscles being used in a golf swing will develop maximum strength—an important attribute in many sport activities." [21]

7. Isometric or static exercises may be used as part of conditioning for space and flight travelers. In space travel, the travelers must cope with the deteriorating effects of weightlessness. Isometric exercise can be performed in the close confines of a spaceship.

8. There is not enough research to support the contention that isometric exercises are dangerous to the cardiovascular system. Dr. Richard Kerber, M.D., conducted an experiment with isometric exercise and concluded, "It appears that in many coronary patients isometric exercise is not as hazardous (in terms of inducing ischemia or arrhythmia) as has been believed." [22]

Consumer Guide® Rating:

1. Isometric exercises are to be considered a possible supplement to a complete fitness program. Under no circumstances should they be viewed as a total fitness program.

2. If isometric exercises are to be used as part of a fitness program, they should be viewed as a means of improving strength and increasing muscle definition or tone. It is recommended that the isometric exercises be supplemented

with isotonic exercises such as flexibility calisthenics (yoga type) and weight training. Aerobic type exercises are also a must.

3. Flexibility and cardiovascular exercises are to be given priority over isometric exercises.

4. Even though the research is still not absolutely conclusive, people suffering from heart disease or high blood pressure should not engage in these exercises unless given permission to do so by a physician knowledgeable in exercise and fitness.

5. Isometric exercises may be useful in improving strength in selected sports by simulating various positions used in the sport, i.e., a golf swing, tennis swing, etc.

6. Isometric exercises may be useful to people who must sit for extended periods of time—on a train, bus, car, or in an airplane.

Thus, isometric exercises must be given a poor rating for the average fitness enthusiast. They are not as effective as calisthenics and cannot be recommended for people who have coronary problems. They can prove beneficial, however, in orthopedic rehabilitation.

ISOTONIC EXERCISE

Isotonic exercise is exercise that requires movement to create muscle contractions. In this discussion, isotonic exercise will refer to training with weights.

The terms "weight training" and "weight lifting" are often used interchangeably, but they are two different things.

Weight training refers to the process of developing muscular strength and/or endurance by exercising with weights or resistive devices. Weight training is based upon the principle that the body adapts to stresses placed upon it, called overload, generally by an overcompensation. By progressively increasing the intensity of effort, you can effect a series of compensatory readjustments and thereby gain in strength and/or endurance.

Weight lifting is a competitive sport, the object of which is to lift, in three basic formats, a greater total poundage than your opponents. These formats, usually referred to as the Olympic lifts because they are the ones used in the Olympic Games, are the press, the snatch, and the clean and jerk. Each is governed by strict performance codes applied by judges.

Body building is another application of weight training—with primary emphasis placed upon the aesthetic aspects of the human torso.

The groundwork for weight training as we know it today was established in the work of Dr. Thomas DeLorme, M.D.[23] The DeLorme method basically consisted of determining by trial and error the most weight that an individual could lift ten times. This was called "10 repetitions maximum" (10 RM). The exerciser then performed sets or bouts of ten repetitions each, the first with half the 10-RM weight, the second with three quarters of the maximum, and the last with 10 RMs.

Most popular weight training programs are based on the three-set, ten-repetition procedure. Modifications are usually in the total number of repetitions performed. Dr. Richard Berger, Ph.D., studied the variations of resistance and repetitions and reported that six repetitions in three bouts yielded the greatest strength gains.[24] Other researchers and investigators state that one set of five to fifteen repetitions performed at maximum effort is sufficient for an exercise period.[25] In the Oxford Technique, ten sets are performed, each consisting of 10 repetitions. "The first set consists of a full 10 RM, and the resistance for each successive set is reduced so that ten repetitions may be completed. The basic principle is to keep the muscles working against maximum resistance even though performance capacity is being reduced by fatigue."[26]

Among the most popular weight lifting programs are Bob Hoffman's *York Barbell and Dumbbell System,*[27] and Weider's *"Triple Progressive" Muscle Building Courses,* by Joe Weider.[28] The average fitness enthusiast is generally dismayed by these programs' tremendous concentration on building of muscle bulk. More suitable for the average exerciser are the *Complete Weight Training Book* by Bill Reynolds,[29] and the *President's Council on Physical Fitness and Sports—Weight Training Program for Strength and Power.*[30] Other acceptable books are *Sports Illustrated's Training with Weights,* [31] Lou Ravelle's *Bodybuilding for Everyone,* [32] and Eric Taylor's *Strength and Stamina Training.*[33]

CRITICISMS OF WEIGHT TRAINING

1. The major criticism of weight training is that it does not develop cardiovascular fitness. Its contribution is in the area of muscle strength and muscle endurance, two of the lesser components of physical fitness.

2. If a person trains incorrectly (doesn't move the weights or doesn't do the exercises throughout the full range of motion), he or she may lose some flexibility.[34] This produces the so-called muscle-bound appearance.

3. One handbook on fitness points out, "Participation in weight training does little, if anything, to develop increased coordination, timing, or motor skills." [35]

4. Lifting weights or weight training can cause the valsalva phenomenon, in which holding the breath during heavy exercise creates excess pressure in the chest cavity. This pressure pushes against the large veins returning blood to the heart. The sudden change in blood pressure and the body's attempt to compensate results in a fluctuation of blood pressure and pulse rate that can result in decreased blood flow to the brain—resulting in dizziness and fainting.[36]

5. Weight training, as a form of static exercise, can cause

"weight lifters' hypertension." This may not be a serious consequence unless the lifter suffers from some heart or brain blood vessel weakness—in other words, aneurysm.[37]

6. Improper lifting can cause back injuries, e.g., herniated discs.[38]

7. Dr. David H. Clarke, Ph.D., professor of physical education at the University of Maryland, says that "high risk cardiovascular patients or people with any overt signs of cardiovascular disease should not lift or should have medical clearance prior to lifting. That is because they may start to demonstrate some cardiac abnormalities."

8. It has been reported that deep knee bends with weights can cause an excessive stretching of the knee ligaments, which would predispose a person to knee injuries.[39]

REBUTTALS

1. Dr. Benjamin H. Massey, Ph.D., and his associates question the use of the term "muscle-bound" and believe it is wrongly associated with weight lifting. "Many of the early professional lifters were extremely strong men, but reputedly were poorly coordinated and of awkward movement. Persons noting this, of course, attributed it to weight lifting." He blames athletic coaches, too, for misusing the term by using it to refer to well-developed boys who were not especially skilled in sports.[40]

2. If safety precautions are taken, the chance of injury in weight lifting is very remote. The late Dr. Peter V. Karpovich, M.D., surveying 111 YMCAs, 5 private clubs, 5 colleges, and 1 high school and reporting on 31,702 weight lifters for 1949–50, found a 1.5-percent incidence of injuries (a total of 494). Most of the injuries consisted of "pulled" muscles or tendons, with back injuries most numerous (100 injuries). Wrists were second with 96, and shoulders third with 77. The incidence of hernias was only five, and only one

death occurred (a barbell falling on a head).[41] Despite the limitations of surveys as a research method, it does appear that weight lifting is not as dangerous as is feared by many people.

3. Contributions of weight training to fitness are many, depending, of course, upon the exercises used and the training procedures followed. According to Dr. Massey, "One can expect from the typical weight-training program ... enlargements of muscles exercised; an increase in muscular efficiency in terms of strength, speed, and power; increased bodily flexibility, especially in the trunk-hip region; improvement in physique; a feeling of relaxation and release from tension; and a sense of fitness and well-being." [42]

4. Dr. Massey states that weight training will not be harmful to a normal, healthy cardiovascular system. He does add, however, that "weight lifting, or for that matter any other vigorous physical effort involving relatively static contraction of the muscles, such as moving a piano, markedly elevates the blood pressure, and may cause a circulatory system weakened by disease to be further injured." [43]

Consumer Guide ®Rating:

1. For development of strength, weight training is perhaps the best approach—either lifting of weights or multi-station gyms such as the *Universal Gym, Nautilus,* etc.

2. Muscle endurance of specific muscles can be developed effectively through weight training.

3. If proper precautions are taken with respect to breathing, adjusting weights properly, and doing the exercises properly, the incidence of injuries in weight training should be quite low.

4. People who have a high coronary risk or cardiovascular disease should not engage in weight training exercises.

5. It is not necessary for the average adult to engage in weight training to develop adequate muscle strength and

muscle endurance; calisthenics can fulfill this need. However, it can help you to improve your strength substantially for better participation in sports.

6. For the average adult male or female interested in developing the physique (broader shoulders, larger chest, better developed calves and thighs, etc.), weight training is unsurpassed and should be considered as an adjunct to a cardiovascular and flexibility program.

7. Weight training should be part of any program for young teen-agers participating in sports, provided the strength work does not predominate over flexibility and cardiovascular training. *Consumer Guide®* agrees with Dr. Benjamin Massey, Ph.D., who stresses the great value of strength in sports, yet adds, "The only precaution that athletes should observe in the use of weights is to limit their use during the season of participation in the sport. Indiscriminate weight training added to the conditioning program outlined by a coach will result in chronic fatigue. . . . Athletes should consult their coach before starting an additional exercise program on their own." [44]

Weight training is, therefore, a good means of improving strength and physique, to be used only as an adjunct to a cardiovascular and flexibility program. Although isotonic exercise (weight training) must be considered poor as general fitness training, it carries a good rating for improvement of muscle strength.

ISOKINETIC EXERCISE

Isokinetic exercise combines isometric and isotonic (progressive resistance) exercises. It involves maximum effort as an isometric exercise, but is carried out through a complete range of motion. This requires a special piece of equipment, a mechanism that controls the amount of resistance you are working against. [45]

An isokinetic machine is one which controls the resistance against which you are working. At a very slow speed, there is no resistance. But when you start to increase exertion, greater resistance is experienced. The machine adapts automatically to the amount of effort being exerted. "By allowing the body to work hard in those positions where the body is structured to do hard work, and to ease off in those positions where the skeletal-muscular system is weak, the isokinetic principle permits an intensive workout with remarkably little danger of injury. That feature of isokinetics is called *accommodating resistance.*"[46]

In isokinetic exercise, excessive strain is automatically (mechanically) taken off the arms and legs at the points of greatest strain. A person doing isokinetic exercise can actually do more muscular work at a higher rate because he or she pushes right past the body's weak points with nary a pause.

Scientific tests conducted on isokinetic exercise indicate that it can be an excellent method of improving strength. One study reported on work with sixty people in three exercise groups. At the end of an eight-week period of exercise, the isokinetic group showed a 35.4-percent increase in total work ability. The increase for the progressive resistance (isotonic) exercise group was 27.5 percent, and for the isometric group only 9.2 percent. Furthermore, in peak force ability, the isokinetic group rose 47.2 percent; the progressive resistance group, 28.6 percent; and the isometric group, 12.1 percent.[47]

Recent work by Doctors Thomas V. Pipes and Jack H. Wilmore of the University of California, Davis, California, supported the superiority of isokinetic exercise over isotonic exercise relative to strength, anthropometric measures, and motor tasks.[48] It may take several years to establish conclusively that isokinetic exercise surpasses isometric and isotonic, but the limited evidence now available indicates that it does.

Technically "pure" isokinetic devices are quite expensive and not designed for home use. They are used primarily for rehabilitative purposes. However, the *Exer-Genie* and similar home devices are modeled on the isokinetic principle of exercise.

EXER-GENIE, APOLLO EXERCISER, AND EXER-GYM

The *Exer-Genie, Apollo Exerciser,* and *Exer-Gym* are evaluated as exercise equipment in a later chapter. They are discussed here, too, due to their popularity and their specific programs and claims.

A kit generally includes the exercise device, an instructional booklet, carrying case, the handles, a foot board, and assorted materials. Optional materials may be purchased—a cassette, workout charts, and additional nylon cord and straps.

The design is similar for all three. At the top of a shaft enclosed in a casing is a metal loop or eye. A nylon line leads out of the shaft through the loop; a handle is attached to each of the two ends of the line. Resistance, preset by revolving the casing around the shaft, is achieved by friction from the movement of the specially braided line winding around the shaft. It can be varied from free movement through maximum effort for individual exercises. The amount of line passing over the shaft determines the approximate resistance in pounds pull, indicated on the calibrated chart which reflects an average resistance in sample testing.

Various exercises are suggested for development of the parts of the body. Attention is generally focused on the legs, upper body, upper third, middle third, and lower third of the body. Provision is usually made for some type of conditioning in which the exerciser runs against resistance.

The *Exer-Genie* program, for example, is a six-minute program of general conditioning that combines a series of exercises called the "Big Four" with two additional exercises—the bicycle and row. The program is to be done daily. The kit recommends that the Big Four be repeated four times, pausing a minute or two between repetitions until breathing is normal and the pulse rate drops to 120.

The Big Four exercises begin with a ten-second isometric hold obtained by applying finger pressure on a nylon cord looped over the handle of the exercise device. The preset resistance is constant as long as no other pressure is placed against the rope. But when strong pressure is applied against it, as in pressing it against the handle with the finger, the rope becomes impossible to move, regardless of the preset resistance. Following the isometric hold, finger pressure is released gradually and the following exercises are performed in sequence: the dead lift, leg press, biceps curl or upright roll, and the standing press.

Following the Big Four, one more minute of additional exercise completes the six-minute program. This is either the bicycling or rowing exercise and is alternated daily. The bicycling exercise is for the legs and derriere, and the rowing exercise is for the shoulders, upper back, and abdominals.

CRITICISMS

1. The major disadvantage of the isokinetic program is that it fails to offer enough cardiovascular endurance development. An evaluation by Dr. Harry D. Olree, Ed.D., at Harding College concluded that "isometric and isotonic training on the Exer-Genie gave negligible increases in cardio-respiratory fitness." [49]

2. Frank Vitale observed in his work that there is some difficulty in controlling and measuring resistance. This makes it difficult to keep a precise record of progress and develop

the techniques.[50] Dr. David H. Clarke, Ph.D., professor of physical education at the University of Maryland, agrees with Mr. Vitale. He says that "although these commercial isokinetic devices have a way of modifying tension, it is a little difficult to know exactly how much tension is programmed into the product. This can present some problems." Dr. Richard Berger, Ph.D., professor of physical education at Temple University, has stated, "It is difficult with these products to allow users to record accurately where they are and what kind of improvement they achieve. This is especially true with young athletes."

3. A third criticism, also issued by Mr. Vitale, is that some people believe that they have not had a long enough workout with the isokinetic devices.[51] This is a subjective judgment and may or may not be a valid criticism.

4. Advertising for *Apollo, Exer-Genie, Exer-Gym,* etc., has implied that the product is a complete fitness program—it improves cardio-respiratory fitness, flexibility, muscle endurance and muscle strength, etc. It is important to understand that this advertising is misleading. Isokinetic devices can make a contribution to muscle strength and muscle endurance, but they are not complete devices and they do not improve cardio-respiratory fitness. Some manufacturers have tried to get around this criticism by adding exercises in which you strain against the rope while running, thereby improving cardio-respiratory fitness through the use of the device. These exercises don't make sense, however; the running in place can be done without the rope.

REBUTTAL

Frank Vitale's list of reasons for using an isokinetic device is a good summary:

1 / Muscle groups can be initially isolated and worked by a variety of special exercises.

2 / Exercises can be adapted from highly sophisticated weight training equipment or barbell training equipment and simulated with the device.

3 / Specific body conditioning for various sports techniques can be combined with technique training, since the various movements can be simulated and performed under controlled resistance.

4 / The equipment is relatively less expensive than weight training equipment, much more easily stored and carried, and can be set up and used anywhere.

5 / The time needed for a complete exercise routine comparable to weight training is considerably less.

6 / It combines the advantages of maximum strength development for isometric contractions with the range of motion that weight training provides, but with the added benefit of maintaining a steady resistance throughout the entire range of movement.[52]

Consumer Guide® Rating: The major shortcoming of the isokinetic device is its lack regarding cardio-respiratory fitness. It does have the definite advantage over isometric exercise of working the muscle through the full range of motion. And it is less expensive than weight training equipment. The fact is, however, that exercise equipment is not necessary to improve muscle strength and muscle endurance. As Dr. Berger has observed, "It doesn't matter whether you overload with weights, with an isokinetic device, through isometrics, or calisthenics. The important thing is to overload the muscles."

If you like to work with equipment, such devices are satisfactory products. But the isokinetic apparatus does not tell you how much resistance you are applying; the figures on the cylinder are estimates.

Consumer Guide® sees the development of specific strengths for sports as the major contribution of isokinetic devices. The user can assume a selected position and then exert to strengthen particular muscles. For example, a javelin thrower interested in improving strength and power can assume the exact position used for releasing the javelin and exert against the device. Or the football kicker can arrange the body in the position in which the greatest amount of power is needed and exert against the device, thereby strengthening the appropriate muscles.

The isokinetic device is good for training athletes and for developing muscle strength, but its contribution to adult fitness programs must be rated poor since it contributes little to cardiovascular and flexibility fitness. Under no circumstances is it to be construed as a complete fitness package or program.

14

FITNESS WITH A TWIST

EVERYONE WANTS YOUR ATTENTION. IN FITNESS IT IS NO different. All types of gimmicks are used—some legitimate and others questionable—to get you to buy a book about your particular fitness problem. *Consumer Guide*® focuses in this chapter on three popular pitches—exercise for the office, exercise to lose weight, and exercise for senior citizens.

FITNESS IN THE BUSINESS WORLD

Who needs exercise more than the desk-bound executive, secretary, engineer, clerk, etc.? Such jobs, requiring the individual to sit at a desk for eight or more hours a day, are the ultimate in sedentary living. A number of exercise programs have been devised for the desk set, most of them combining traditional approaches to fitness with a smattering of cardiovascular exercise.

ROBERT R. SPACKMAN: EXERCISE IN THE OFFICE

Exercise in the Office was written by Robert R. Spackman, a registered physical therapist and the head athletic trainer at

Southern Illinois University, to help office workers develop "muscle strength, circulation, and flexibility." [1] Spackman specifically points out that the program does not emphasize cardiovascular fitness, nor is it a weight-reducing program: "There are a few cardiovascular exercises such as skipping rope, running in place, running up and down stairs, and jogging or running. The effectiveness of this depends on how often you run or skip rope, and how much you put into your program. Any of the above will increase your endurance and improve your cardiovascular system." [2]

The Spackman program consists of a series of exercise routines for selected areas of the body: neck and shoulders, shoulders and upper back, arms and upper back, chest, lower back, abdomen, hips and buttocks, knees and legs, feet and ankles.

Consumer Guide® Rating: A series of good muscle strength and flexibility exercises that can be done in an office, Spackman's program falls short as a complete exercise plan. As Spackman himself acknowledges, it includes very little cardiovascular work. Another major drawback to the program is that there is no specified progression of exercise. The plan is rated poor as an overall fitness program.

OTTO GRAHAM AND CARL W. SELIN: PHYSICAL FITNESS FOR THE BUSINESS MAN

Otto Graham, director of athletics, and Carl W. Selin, head of the department of physical education—both at the U.S. Coast Guard Academy—wrote *Physical Fitness for the Business Man* for the modern executive.[3] They believe that a person following their program can expect to look better, feel better, and work better; and reduce weight control problems; increase the efficiency of the heart, circulatory system, respiratory system; be less vulnerable to tension and stress; and have increased muscle strength, endurance, and flexibility. Their basic conditioning program consists of eight exercises for the major areas of the body: legs, waist, abdomen, arms and shoulders, back, and cardio-respiratory system. The first seven exercises are designed primarily for the major muscle groups of the body; the last is a five- to ten-minute endurance exercise that may be a continuous run-jog, a swim, running in place, or bench stepping.

The authors suggest fifteen substitute exercises the exerciser may prefer to the eight recommended ones, eleven resistance exercises used with weights, and a set of isometric exercises.

Consumer Guide® Rating: A somewhat dated program, the Graham-Selin plan recommends a number of questionable exercises, e.g., squat thrusts, the body arch, the alternate toe touch, and the back raiser. Several of the weight-training exercises are also potentially dangerous. The five to ten minutes of distance workout is, of course, too short for cardiovascular training value and should be at least fifteen minutes.

Graham and Selin do give some good advice on how to begin distance endurance exercise, and the program is progressive. But they come up short when they recommend a half-mile of running for people over forty-one years of age and one mile for those twenty-six to forty-one years old; a recommendation of one-and-a-half to two miles for all age groups would be more appropriate. The program is rated as marginal.

WEIGHT CONTROL THROUGH EXERCISE

Up until a few years ago, not much was being written about exercise and weight control. The emphasis was on diet. In the late 1960s and early '70s, many began to look upon exercise as a supplement to diet programs. Today, interest seems to have shifted to exercise, with diet playing a support role. Dr. Fredrick Stare, M.D., a world-famous nutritionist, has noted that "The talk used to be all 'diet and exercise.' Today it's exercise and diet." [4] Stare goes on to note that "recent studies of obesity at Harvard's School of Public Health quite clearly indicate that most people who are overweight are not that way simply because they consume too many calories, but rather because of lethargy and the lack of exercise." [5]

The relationship of physical activity to weight control was discussed in an earlier chapter. The important thing to remember is that the best physical activities for controlling body weight are big-muscle activities such as walking, cycling, swimming, and jogging (at least four times a week).

RICHARD L. HITTLEMAN: WEIGHT CONTROL THROUGH YOGA

In *Weight Control Through Yoga,* Richard L. Hittleman contends that he has had as much experience with the problem of obesity as any person in the United States and that his is therefore "the plan that has been tested the most extensively and found to be the most successful." [6] He claims that his special combination of yoga exercises and yoga principles of nutrition results in a drastic loss and redistribution of weight and firming of flabby areas for all overweight people.

Hittleman's book is divided into three sections: the yoga theory of weight regulation, the optional fasting plan, and the exercise routines. *Consumer Guide®* will focus on the first and last parts. An evaluation of the fasting plan can be found in the *Consumer Guide® Rating the Diets.*

Hittleman's primary thesis is this:

Permanent regulation and control of weight must be natural by-products of the total way in which one lives!

Instead of attempting to graft various plans for weight control onto an existing mode of life, the most practical and successful solution to the problem is to alter the way of life. It is possible to undertake a manner of living in which weight regulation and permanent control are inevitable; wherein, among many other positive things, "exercising" is looked forward to as one of the most enjoyable activities of the day and "dieting" harbors no sense of denial or restriction. Yoga is just such a total way of life.[7]

With that as his guiding principle, he then provides three yoga "routines." Each is to serve as one day's practice and cover four essential aspects of weight loss: reducing, firming, stimulating organs and glands, and controlling mind and emotions (see Figure 32).

FIGURE 32 / SAMPLE HITTLEMAN YOGA
WEIGHT-CONTROL ROUTINES

	ROUTINE 1	ROUTINE 2	ROUTINE 3
Reducing	Complete Breath	Complete Breath	Complete Breath
	Side Bend	Triangle	Rishi's Posture
	Cobra	Twist	Dancer's Posture
	Bow	Leg Over	Roll Twist
	Lie Down; Sit Up	Chin Exercise	Seated Side Bend
Firming	Leg Clasp	Back Stretch	Lion
	Side Raise	Shoulder Raise	Alternate Leg Pull
		Locust	Back Push-Up
Stimulating organs and glands	Abdominal Exercises	Head Stand	Shoulder Stand
Controlling mind and emotions	Direction of the Life-Force	Alternate Nostril Breathing	Deep Relaxation

---

Richard L. Hittleman, *Weight Control Through Yoga.* NY: Bantam Books, 1974, p. 39.

Hittleman provides a Stage A, Stage B, and Stage C for the three yoga routines. The A movements are the most elementary. This is the beginning stage of the program, when you are heaviest. The B positions are intermediate movements for use when you have lost approximately half of your intended weight loss. Stage C consists of advanced movements for use when you are approximately five to ten pounds from your final goal. You can also use Stage C as a maintenance program.

Consumer Guide® Rating: *Consumer Guide®* agrees with Hittleman that to be successful in losing weight you must change your way of life. We do not feel, however, that yoga is the best means.

Research has shown that yoga exercise consumes relatively few calories—about 200 per hour [8]—which is not much. For most people, yoga exercise is not especially effective in controlling body weight. The exception may be the person who is only slightly out of caloric balance and who might substitute one hour of yoga exercise for an hour of sleeping or sitting. In that case, ten to fifteen pounds might be lost in one year. Some yoga exercises can be helpful in firming up particular muscles but not in reducing the percentage of fat on the body. To reduce body fat, you must go into caloric deficit, preferably through large-muscle activity.

Many of the book's statements on weight control are erroneous. The assertion that raising the legs above the head and using a shoulder stand stimulates the thyroid gland is a dubious claim; *Consumer Guide®* finds no evidence to support this notion. And we cannot recommend the practice of fasting.[9] *Weight Control Through Yoga* is not recommended.

FRANK KONISHI: EXERCISE EQUIVALENTS OF FOOD

Frank Konishi is professor of nutrition at Southern Illinois University. In *Exercise Equivalents of Food,* he relates exercise to calories directly, by listing the exercise equivalents of over six hundred common foods (using the average energy cost of walking, bicycling, stepping, swimming, and jogging).[10]

Consumer Guide® Rating: A valuable book with good information about the energy equivalents of selected foods, *Exercise Equivalents of Food* receives no rating because it provides no exercise program.

GRANT GWINUP: ENERGETICS: YOUR KEY TO WEIGHT CONTROL

Dr. Grant Gwinup, M.D., sets out in *Energetics: Your Key to Weight Control,* to show the relationship of physical activity to weight control.[11] He gives all kinds of information on how big a problem weight control is, the types of food we eat, basal metabolic rate, where fat is, why we get hungry, the basic cause of obesity, frauds in controlling body weight, and how to lose weight.

His program is methodical in concept. First you find out how many calories you burn off every day. To do this, you keep track of every bite you eat and your hour-by-hour activities for one week (a week when you are neither gaining nor losing weight). Using the charts at the end of his book to calculate calorie intake and use, you next subtract your activity calories from your food calories. According to Gwinup, the difference will be 500 to 2,000 calories. After doing this every day for a week, you will have a fairly accurate average "baseline expenditure figure." Now you begin to fill out an energy balance sheet daily. You count your calorie intake and enter it under "credits." Under "debits" you write in your baseline expenditure, plus that day's count for activities and exercise.[12]

Consumer Guide® Rating: Although a book with excellent information on exercise and weight, *Energetics* provides no exercise plan. The reader is simply told to be more active. Consequently, *Energetics* receives no rating.

SENIOR CITIZENS

Only recently have fitness leaders and directors focused attention on senior citizens. With current research strongly suggesting that exercise may slow the symptoms of aging, more and more people recognize exercise as essential for the health of senior citizens. Their fitness needs are largely identical to those of the average citizen, although it may take more time to make improvements. When there has been neglect of exercise, it takes time to get back in shape. Research clearly indicates that elderly people who are active have more productive lives.

FRANCES KING: GOLDEN AGE EXERCISES

Golden Age Exercises was written by Frances King.[13] King, trained in physical education and working at a day center with people who were sixty years old or more (average age seventy-nine), devised a series of exercises for senior citizens. The series includes four sets: finger, hand, and arm exercises; followed by shoulder, chest, and neck; then shoulders, abdomen, hips, and back; and, in the last chapter, leg exercises. Most of the exercises are excellent for older people.

Consumer Guide® Rating: The major shortcoming is that King does not have a plan of progression. The older person is told to do each exercise approximately three to five times, with no adjustments made for improvement. Furthermore, no cardiovascular improvement exercises are given. Nor is there any attempt to point out which exercises are best. With over eighty exercises listed and no comparisons made, the program becomes unmanageable. A few exercises are potentially hazardous. Consequently, *Golden Age Exercises* is rated as a poor fitness program.

HERBERT A. deVRIES: VIGOR REGAINED

Dr. Herbert A. deVries, Ph.D., has written a home exercise program for senior citizens. *Vigor Regained* is based on the study of the 112 men who participated in his fitness program at the Center for Aging Research at the University of Southern California.[14] According to deVries, the enjoyment of old age depends largely on one's physical condition. His aim is to help the sedentary out-of-shape older person regain a state of positive good health—not just absence of disease, but a feeling of physical well-being and vigor.

Dr. deVries is careful to warn against the dangers of exercise: "Even the conditioning program itself, if unplanned and uncontrolled, can constitute a hazard, especially in the presence of unrecognized heart disease." [15] His program takes into account such individual factors as age, fitness level, type and rate of exercise, and heart rate response. He strongly emphasizes the principle of gradual progression, starting out at an easy level and building up slowly.

First deVries recommends obtaining your doctor's approval for the conditioning program. Only then do you move on to the chapter on self-testing and self-monitoring. With the self-testing you determine your capacity for exercise; self-monitoring measures your response to each activity. Because both testing and monitoring require measuring your heart rate (pulse rate), the reader is taught this procedure.

You then choose which of the two fitness programs (Level 1 or Level 2) is best. Both programs consist of the same three types of exercise (endurance, calisthenics, and flexibility), differing in intensity. Level 1 is for beginners; Level 2 is for those who are in relatively good shape or who have completed Level 1.

Each exercise session begins with an endurance activity (walking in Level 1, jogging and walking in Level 2). Distance is increased over a period of days. The purpose of this part of the program is to condition the heart, lungs, and blood vessels and to reduce nervous tension.

The calisthenics (for muscle strengthening) and static stretching exercises (for flexibility) are basically the same for both levels, differing mainly in the time spent on each type. Level 2 calisthenics are performed a little faster and stretching exercises are held longer. On the whole, Level 2 takes less time than Level 1. The static stretching exercises are progressive; you work up slowly and comfortably to the ultimate position.

Consumer Guide® Rating: *Vigor Regained* is an excellent program that is a must for anyone who is moving into his or her later years and who is interested in a fitness plan. The principles that deVries outlines are sound and can be used by people of all ages. He provides an adequate warm-up and cool-down. He also provides correct recommendations regarding intensity, duration, and frequency of exercise.

THE PRESIDENT'S COUNCIL: THE FITNESS CHALLENGE ... IN THE LATER YEARS

The President's Council on Physical Fitness and Sports prepared (under the direction of Dr. William Haskell, Ph.D., then program director for the Council) a pamphlet on exercise for older Americans.[16] This program presents three series of exercises graded according to difficulty or amount of stress. These series are identified as the red, the white, and the blue—the blue being the most difficult and sustained.

The first step is to check with a physician for advice. After your physician has reviewed the program and given permission, you proceed with a few simple tests. The first is a walk test to determine how many minutes (up to ten) you can walk briskly, without undue difficulty or discomfort, on a level surface. If you can finish just three minutes, you are to start at the red level. If you can go beyond three minutes but not quite to ten minutes, you spend approximately a week or two at the red level and then move up to the white level. If you can go through the whole ten minutes, you are ready for the second test, the walk/jog test #1.

The walk/jog test #1 consists of alternately walking fifty steps and jogging fifty steps for a total of six minutes. If you can complete the six minutes without any difficulty, you proceed to the blue level. If not, you stay at the white level. Again, if you find this test easy, you can try walk/jog test #2. This one consists of alternately walking one hundred steps and jogging one hundred steps for a total of ten minutes. If you can complete the ten-minute blue test without difficulty, you can probably handle the blue program and might even progress to the President's Council fitness program described in Chapter 11. If you cannot complete the ten-minute walk/jog, you stay at the blue level or even possibly at the white level.

The exercise sessions are to be done every day for approximately thirty minutes. A sample sequence of exercises for the red program includes the following: walking two minutes, doing six exercises, then walking two to five minutes; this is followed by seven minutes of calisthenics and alternately walking fifty steps and jogging ten steps for one to three minutes; the workout is then finished with a walk of one to three minutes. The sequence is to be performed as a continuous activity.

Consumer Guide® Rating: An excellent program, the President's Council *Later Years* plan is sound and progressive. The only objection is to the statement that activity should be increased until it is sustained hard and long enough to keep the pulse rate above 130 for several minutes and to increase body temperature gradually to the point of perspiration. It would have been far better to age-group the pulse rates rather than use a cutoff of 130. For some people, a pulse rate of 105 may be the maximum safe level.

15

HOW YOUR FAVORITE SPORT RATES AS EXERCISE

THE IDEA OF USING A SPORT AS A PRIMARY EXERCISE IS appealing. One fitness expert, Dr. Lawrence Golding, Ph.D., told *Consumer Guide®* in an interview that "the main advantage of sports is the fun element. It is a lot more fun to go out and play a sport than it is to do calisthenics. Furthermore, *some* people thrive on competition, and sport gives them that element. Finally, there is some satisfaction in possessing the skill and displaying the skills. These are strong motivators and important benefits, but they are not fitness benefits."

FACTORS AFFECTING FITNESS BENEFITS

What *can* you get out of your sport? Can you use it to "kill two birds with one stone"—enjoyment and fitness? The answer is not simple. A particular sport may be a super way to become fit or it may be a disaster. And it's not just a matter of selection. Effectiveness depends also on how you play the sport, your skill and fitness level, your competitiveness, and, finally, the potential of the sport for fitness training. Dr. Golding, director of the exercise physiology laboratory and professor of physical education at the University of Nevada, Las Vegas, discussed these points with *Consumer Guide.*®

HOW YOU PLAY THE SPORT

Your approach to the sport makes a big difference. Dr. Golding made the point that most people engage in a sport as recreation with no attention to developing fitness: "I think that the average person goes out and plays tennis at whatever level is possible. But there is no planned progression so that he or she is getting fitter and fitter and can play harder and harder. The problem is there is no kind of progression for most people in sport."

YOUR SKILL LEVEL

A second factor is your skill level. Dr. Golding insists that skill development is essential if sports are to play a meaningful role in building fitness. Casual tennis that consists primarily of walking to pick up the ball, or swimming that is mostly floating, will do little for fitness. For swimming to be effective, for example, you have to systematically swim laps and each time to increase the number.

YOUR FITNESS LEVEL

The third consideration is your fitness level. Dr. Golding says: "I think that when you are not conditioned you only do a little bit and then stop." According to Golding, a big problem with sports for fitness is the fact that most people engage in sporting activities as weekend activities, whereas training requires steady and frequent participation. "Now if you are in a position where you can go cross-country skiing every day and make a training program out of it, just like you would a jogging program, then fine, I think it would be great to do cross-country skiing."

COMPETITION

Some of us are more competitive than others. In Dr. Golding's experience, interest in competition seems to be related to whether or not an individual has had extensive experience with competitive sports in the past. He has found that ex-athletes usually crave competition and nonathletes do not. In work done at Kent State University he found that the 130 businessmen (who were not ex-athletes) found the exercise program attractive because it didn't require much skill and wasn't competitive. "Any competition they got was only with themselves."

On the other hand, competition is important for those who really need it to make a go of fitness. Some find activity for its own sake too dull. Golding regards competition as an individual consideration: "If you're a good tennis player and have success with it, you'll probably continue to play it. But if you had poor experiences with physical activity then the less competitive activities would probably be more desirable for you."

If you enjoy competition, have a favorite sport, have a good skill level, a good fitness level, *and* have the opportunity to participate three or more times a week, you can use sports as a means to achieve fitness. That may be a pretty big order, but adjustments can be made. If your fitness level is not up to par, a reconditioning program (of several months) may reduce this problem. If you find that you have the opportunity to play the sport only on weekends, you can condition your body through other activities during the week to maintain fitness and enjoy participation to its fullest.

There are no pat answers on sports as a primary exercise. You are now aware of the factors. Regularity, rigorousness, and duration are the keys. Engage in your sport three times a week, get your heart rate into the target range, and spend thirty minutes each time, and you will make fitness gains.

HOW THE SPORTS STACK UP

Everyone has a favorite sport. For some it is NFL football, for others frisbee throwing, abalone diving, acrobatics, yachting, or wrist wrestling. The variety is endless.

In this book, of course, *Consumer Guide®* is interested only in participatory sports. This chapter will focus on the activities found to be most popular in a survey by the President's Council on Physical Fitness and Sports—bowling, bicycling, swimming, golf, softball, jogging or running, tennis, volleyball, water skiing, and skiing (downhill and cross-country) [1]—plus a few others that *Consumer Guide®* selected for inclusion (handball/squash/racquetball, basketball, and ice and roller skating).

BASKETBALL

Advantages: Dr. Sam Fox, M.D., former president of the American College of Cardiology and now professor of medicine at Georgetown University, rates basketball as an "excellent endurance-generating exercise." [2] If played regularly three or more times a week, it can condition the heart and lungs. This sport burns a lot of calories (630 to 750+ per hour). [3]

Disadvantages: Doctors David Shepro, Ph.D., and Howard Knuttgen, Ph.D., summarize the disadvantages: "(1) It requires other players; (2) activities such as running, swimming, rowing, are far better CV [cardiovascular] conditioners; and (3) the chances for incurring injury are good, especially for the older participant." [4] According to Dr. Allan Ryan, M.D., editor of *Postgraduate Medicine* and *The Physician and Sportsmedicine,* basketball "is a sport for the already fit. You don't play basketball to get fit; you must be fit to play it." [5]

Additional Comments: Basketball can be enjoyed by and be beneficial to older people, provided they have engaged in the sport for years, they warm up properly before the activity, enjoy competition, understand their limitations, play regularly (three times a week), and are fit!

BICYCLING

Advantages: Bicycling is an excellent activity for practically all age groups. It provides a vigorous workout that conditions the cardiovascular system. Dr. Paul Dudley White emphasized the importance of exercising the leg muscles from childhood on and was convinced that "cycling for all ages is one of the best ways to accomplish and maintain physical fitness." [6] Another advantage is that bicycling is fun, says Dr. John Boyer, M.D.[7]

A third advantage is that bicycling subjects the body to little trauma. The obese, overweight, or very unfit sometimes find that running causes some leg problems. Bicyclists experience a lower incidence of injury due to leg trauma. And cycling is excellent for improving the strength of the leg and back muscles.

Disadvantages: Perhaps the biggest problem with bicycling is the fact that most people pedal too slowly to derive maximum cardiovascular benefit. For the great majority of people, cycling at eight miles an hour will not elicit a target heart rate. If you are going to use bicycling as a primary means of exercise to condition your heart and lungs it will be necessary to pedal fast, ride up hills, or use a gear that offers substantial resistance. An occasional pulse check will tell you if you are working hard enough to produce training. One skeptic adds, "Because the body weight is on the bike, it is less intense than running." [9]

There is also the risk of shortened hamstring muscles on the back of the leg and loss of leg flexibility, related—

according to Dr. Theodore Klumpp, M.D., medical consultant to the President's Council on Physical Fitness and Sports—to the fact that "the pedal at the instep fails to give maximum extension to the ankle and foot." [10] Another disadvantage is that weather can restrict use; ice, snow, and fog can be particularly hazardous.

Additional Comments: Bicycling burns around 350 to 449 calories per hour for the average person.[11] More or fewer calories can be used depending on the speed, the terrain, and the type of bicycle.

BOWLING

Advantages: Bowling is a family-type recreational activity that can be good therapy for the participants. One study polled 260 bowlers and found that 7 out of 8 felt more relaxed after bowling.[12] Another advantage is that since it does not require much exertion, there is no age or body-type limit to participation.

Disadvantages: Bowling does not enhance fitness. All seven of the fitness experts polled by Casey Conrad, Executive Director of the President's Council on Physical Fitness and Sports, agreed that the game does little or nothing to improve physical fitness (see Figure 33).[13] It has been estimated that it takes you about two-and-a-half seconds (if that) to deliver the ball. In each game, you exercise (bowl) less than one minute. A full evening of bowling (three games) gives the average person about three minutes of exercise.

Additional Comments: For the average person, bowling burns about 160 to 190 calories per hour.[14]

Anyone with low back pain should approach the game with caution.

FIGURE 33 / A QUICK SCORECARD ON 14 SPORTS AND EXERCISES

	JOGGING	BICYCLING	SWIMMING	SKATING (ICE OR ROLLER)	HANDBALL/SQUASH	SKIING-NORDIC	SKIING-ALPINE	BASKETBALL	TENNIS	CALISTHENICS	WALKING	GOLF*	SOFTBALL	BOWLING
PHYSICAL FITNESS														
Cardio-respiratory endurance (stamina)	21	19	21	18	19	16	19	16	16	10	13	8	6	5
Muscular endurance	20	18	20	17	19	18	17	16	16	13	14	8	8	5
Muscular strength	17	16	14	15	15	15	15	14	14	16	11	9	7	5
Flexibility	9	9	15	13	16	14	13	14	14	19	7	9	9	7
Balance	17	18	12	20	17	21	16	16	16	15	8	8	7	6
GENERAL WELL-BEING														
Weight control	21	20	15	17	19	15	19	19	16	12	13	6	7	5
Muscle definition	14	15	14	14	11	14	13	13	13	18	11	6	5	5
Digestion	13	12	13	11	13	9	10	12	12	11	11	7	8	7
Sleep	16	15	16	15	15	12	12	11	11	12	14	6	7	6
Total	148	142	140	140	139	134	134	134	128	126	102	66*	64	51

Here's a summary of how seven experts rated various sports and exercises. Ratings are on a scale of 0 to 3, thus a rating of 21 indicates maximum benefit (a score of 3 by all 7 panelists). Ratings were made on the basis of regular (minimum of 4 times per week), vigorous (duration of 30 minutes to one hour per session) participation in each activity.

* Ratings for golf are based on the fact that many Americans use a golf cart and/or caddy. If you walk the links, the physical fitness value moves up appreciably.

Taken from C. C. Conrad, "How Different Sports Rate in Promoting Physical Fitness," *Medical Times*, May, 1976 (Reprint), pp. 4–5.

GOLF

Advantages: Golf has the advantage of getting you outdoors. You will burn more calories than if you just sat for the three to four hours it takes you to play. It also has the advantage of developing camaraderie among friends.

Disadvantages: Shepro and Knuttgen neatly summarize the limitations of golf in fitness training. "Golf is a sport activity of very low intensity. Strength and aerobic fitness are affected to little or no extent. Golf can be employed to use up calories (but is only effective if you don't hit the '19th hole'). Golf carts utilize lots of energy (not the golfer's) but obtain no conditioning effect." [15] Casey Conrad's panel of seven experts came to the same conclusion. Most felt that golf provides little physical benefit in that it does not place a demand on the cardiovascular system.[16]

Additional Comments: Playing in a twosome, carrying your own clubs, and walking briskly burns about 240 to 320 calories an hour. If you use a cart, you burn only 185 to 220 calories in an hour.[17]

George Romney has turned his golf game into a cardiovascular activity. The former Governor of Michigan and U.S. Secretary of Housing and Urban Development hits the ball and then chases after it by running. The result is that he saves time and improves cardiovascular fitness.

HANDBALL/SQUASH/RACQUETBALL

These three sports are lumped together because they feature similar types of action. Generally, handball is the most vigorous of the three, followed by squash and then racquetball, but the level depends upon the individual, the skill level, and the degree of competitiveness.

Advantages: In these sports, all the major muscle groups

of the body are used. If you have a good skill level and are playing against someone of similar ability, good cardiovascular conditioning will take place, although not to the extent experienced in running or swimming.[18] A large number of calories are expended (approximately 650 to 755 per hour).[19]

Disadvantages: Dr. Sam Fox cautions that the "demands on ligaments and joints may cause problems in middle to later years." [20] Here again, as in basketball, you should be fit *before* you begin to participate in these sports. Availability of courts can be another problem.

Additional Comments: Care should be taken to play with individuals of ability equal to yours. This reduces frustration. An adequate warm-up should precede the playing. It is also important to play on a regular basis, avoid injuries, and be sure your body can get enough oxygen while playing.

RUNNING

Advantages: Running is one of the best activities for cardiovascular fitness, body composition, muscle endurance, and strength of the legs (see Chapters 8 and 9). According to Sam Fox, it is "the most efficient and inexpensive approach to enhancing endurance capacity." [21] Dr. Warren Guild, M.D., former president of the American College of Sports Medicine, says that running "can squeeze maximum consistent effort into a minimum amount of time." [22]

It is very easy to regulate running. You can adjust your load to your fitness level without fear of overdoing it. According to Kenneth Cooper, running is the best of the big four cardiovascular exercises—running, swimming, bicycling, walking—in that order.[23]

A significant number of calories are burned in a relatively short period of time—approximately 585 to 700 calories per hour, more or less depending upon the speed.[24]

Disadvantages: Running does little to improve muscle

strength, particularly in the upper body. Furthermore, the middle third musculature of the body does not benefit by this exercise. Running may shorten the muscles in the back of the leg, thereby reducing flexibility and making you more prone to injury and leg pain.

Running is not for everyone. The endomorph (the heavy person) may find the activity too traumatic to legs, ankles, and knees. The highly unfit or deconditioned person will experience similar problems.

Additional Comments: Running sessions must be preceded with warm-ups, and a running regimen should begin with a "starter" program of walk-jog alternates.[25]

An excellent book on running is *The Complete Book of Running*,* by James F. Fixx. It is a best seller that deserves its reputation. It just may be the best book on running to date. *Running* tells you like it is about running. The whys, hows, problems, and joys of running are explored by a writer who apparently writes what he lives. Fixx recommends using pulse rate as your guide and listening to your body as you run and make improvements. Good, sound advice.

SKATING (ICE/ROLLER)

Advantages: Both types of skating are good for improving cardiovascular fitness. According to the *Physical Fitness Encyclopedia,* skating is an excellent exercise: "The major muscle groups of the body, such as the legs and arms, get an excellent workout because of these vigorous movements. The lungs and heart also get a good workout if the skating is strenuous enough. If the skating is done vigorously, you'll burn calories and increase circulo-respiratory endurance."[26] Since these sports burn 295 to 350 calories (leisurely skating) or 520 to 620 calories (skating vigorously),[27] they can play a significant role in weight control.

---

* J. F. Fixx, *The Complete Book of Running.* NY: Random House, 1977.

Disadvantages: Dr. Evalyn S. Gendel, M.D., has made the point that the skills necessary to skate well are not easily learned in adulthood; most skaters learned early in life.[28] Another potential obstacle is lack of facilities. A drawback to skating as a fitness enhancer is the low demand on strength and muscle endurance.

SKIING (DOWNHILL)

Advantages: Some fitness experts (Doctors Larry Lamb, M.D.; Hans Kraus, M.D.; Theodore Klumpp, M.D.; and Evalyn Gendel, M.D.) assert that downhill skiing can be a good endurance activity.[29] Others (Doctors Allan Ryan, M.D.; David Shepro, Ph.D.; and Howard Knuttgen, Ph.D.) believe that the contribution of downhill skiing to cardiovascular fitness is extremely limited.[30] Short runs probably make little contribution to cardiovascular fitness whereas longer runs of ten minutes or more may make a significant cardiovascular contribution.

Disadvantages: This is another activity for the fit. Dr. Hans Kraus insists, "It is especially important to have good basic muscular fitness; otherwise there is great exposure to injury." [31]

If you could ski downhill for one hour nonstop, you would burn 500 to 590 calories.[32] Most people don't; they ski for five minutes or so, stop, and then take the lift back up, defeating the continuity of the exercise.

Additional Comments: Because the sport is anaerobic (involving intense oxygen demand) at times and because of the need for good muscular fitness, preconditioning classes should be engaged in six to eight weeks prior to actual skiing. Furthermore, because of the cold air and rigorousness of the activity, a proper warm-up should precede each session. Anyone with a history of knee trouble should definitely spend several months conditioning the thighs to reduce the chances of reinjuring the knee.[33]

SKIING (CROSS-COUNTRY)

Advantages: Shepro and Knuttgen are enthusiastic supporters of this sport: "Cross-country skiing (performed with vigor!) constitutes one of the best forms of activity for cardiovascular fitness. A very large portion of the body muscle mass is called upon to perform heavy exercise for extended periods." [34]

Cross-country skiing is far less expensive than downhill skiing and can be enjoyed by practically anyone. Hills are not necessary, and preliminaries are minimal; one half-hour of instruction is enough preparation to start you off with a reasonable degree of proficiency.

This is a very high energy-consumption activity. Up to 1,000 calories an hour can be burned. [35]

Disadvantages: A minimum amount of muscular fitness is desirable (although not as much as you would need for downhill skiing).

Additional Comments: Because of the high intensity of this sport, it is best to start out slowly.

Simply stated, cross-country skiing is a superb fitness activity. Many of the fitness components can be improved, including circulo-respiratory endurance, body composition, muscle strength, muscle endurance, and flexibility.

SOFTBALL

Advantages: Softball is a pleasant activity and enjoyable recreation for many people. Playing softball burns around 250 to 280 calories per hour. [36]

Disadvantages: Softball scores very low on the fitness scale. The consensus of most experts is that too much time is spent sitting around doing nothing. Warren Guild, M.D., and Theodore Klumpp, M.D., Hans Kraus, M.D., and Allan Ryan, M.D., all feel that the game makes little contribution to any of the fitness components. Also, it takes a number of people to play the game.[37]

SWIMMING

Advantages: Swimming is one of the best fitness activities around. The heart and lungs shift into heightened action, the legs and arms are used continuously and rhythmically, the back and abdominal muscles are strengthened, and swimming is relaxing.[38]

Another advantage, emphasized by Warren Guild, is that it is a "nonweight-bearing sport; it's good for people recovering from hip, knee, and ankle problems." [39] Dr. Sam Fox values swimming ability as a safety essential—to reduce the incidence of drowning deaths.[40]

Swimming is an excellent activity for burning calories; a swimmer uses 350 to 420 calories per hour, and more if the swimming is fast. It is particularly good for the overweight in that a lot of calories are burned without risking trauma to the legs; the water supports body weight.

Disadvantages: The two biggest potential obstacles are not knowing how to swim and having no access to a pool or body of water.

Additional Comments: Fitness benefits from swimming occur only if you swim actively. Paddling around in the pool or resting on a raft or a lounge chair does not qualify. You have to move to improve. The swimming should cover about thirty yards a minute or more, and target heart rates must be reached to make fitness improvements.

TENNIS

Advantages: Dr. Sam Fox approves of tennis for fitness: "Excellent for body shaping, flexibility and balance; stimulates endurance if vigorously played." [41] The key words are "if vigorously played." Too many people play tennis in a way that does little to condition the heart and lungs. This is particularly true of beginners.

Shepro and Knuttgen are only lukewarm: "Tennis is predominantly an anaerobic activity with quick movements and short sprints mixed with rather long recovery periods. While not considered to be a cardiovascular conditioner, tennis played by skilled players and involving extended rallies can make a meaningful, although not great, contribution in this respect." [42]

Disadvantages: Dr. Evalyn Gendel, for one, is concerned about the anxiety levels generated by tennis and other sports; people worry too much about their game.[43]

The biggest disadvantage is the high level of ability necessary to get a good workout. Continuous play requires volleying back and forth, which is necessary for this sport to have a training effect on the cardiovascular system. Constantly stopping to serve or retrieve the ball stops play and reduces the contribution of the sport to fitness.

Other disadvantages are the need for a partner and court. The current tennis boom, however, seems to be alleviating these two problems.

VOLLEYBALL

Advantages: Volleyball is an uncomplicated game that can be enjoyed by people of many ages and skill levels. It is not difficult to learn. A good point is made by Sam Fox: "Volleyball is less demanding than basketball and it can be easier to organize teams with odd numbers and with less equal skills than with basketball." [44]

Disadvantages: Marshall L. Walters writes in the *Physical Fitness Encyclopedia* that "the value of volleyball for physical fitness ranges from near 0 to 100. The degree of fitness obtained is dependent upon the training program and the level of volleyball played." [45] According to Marshall, the casual volleyball game produces few physical fitness benefits. Volleyball is a fitness-effective program only at the upper levels of competition.

The necessity for others players is a problem, although not as critical as in basketball. Volleyball is another sport in which fitness training does not take place unless your skill level and the ability of your opponents are quite good.

WATER SKIING

Advantages: According to Dr. Carlton R. Meyers, Ed.D., water skiing can make an important contribution to physical fitness, especially in muscular strength and endurance. The potential contribution to cardio-respiratory endurance is less predictable and depends upon the work load and the existing fitness level of the participant. "The work load is determined by (1) the length of the period spent in continuous skiing and the total time on a given occasion; (2) the amount of activity entailed; and (3) the type of skiing done." [46]

Disadvantages: Again Carlton Meyers makes an interesting observation: "While the contribution of water skiing to cardio-respiratory endurance appears limited, your level of cardio-respiratory endurance will determine the overall vigor with which you can water ski." [47] In other words, if you start out with a low fitness level you may find your enjoyment of the sport is limited—a distinct disadvantage. Furthermore, Dr. Sam Fox points out that water skiing is "largely isometric, with an anxiety component which makes it not good for heart disease patients." [48]

Additional Comments: To water ski, you should be a swimmer. You should also make sure that your skis are in good repair and are the proper size and you should wear special flotation gear.

SUMMING UP

As a summary, *Consumer Guide*® provides Figures 34 and 35, two tables evaluating the fitness value of a large number of popular sports.

FIGURE 34 / FITNESS BENEFITS OF SELECTED SPORTS

H–High, M–Medium, L–Low, M-H–Depends whether recreation (M) or Vigorous (H)

Sport	C-R Endurance	Muscle Strength				Muscle Endurance				Flexibility			
		Arms	Legs	Abdomen	Back	Arms	Legs	Abdomen	Back	Shoulder	Hip	Elbow	Knee
Australian Football	H	L	H	M	M	M	H	M	M	L	M	L	H
Baseball	L	M	M	L	L-M	L	M	M	M	H	M	H	H
Basketball	H	L	H	L	L	M	H	M	M	M	M	M	H
Bobsledding	L	L	M	L	L	L	L	L	L-M	L	L	L	L
Boxing	H	H	H	H	H	H	H	H	H	L-M	M	H	H
Cross Country Running	H	M	H	M	H	M	H	H	H	L	L	L	H
Cricket	L	L	M	M	M	L	M	M	M	H	M	H	H
Diving	L	L	L	H	L	L	L	L	L	H	H	L	L
Fencing	M-H	M	M-H	M	M	M	M	M	M	M	H	H	H
Field Hockey	H	M	H	M	M	M	H	M	M-H	M	H	H	H
Football													
a. Tackle	H	M-H	H	H	H	M	H	M	H	L	H	L	M
b. Playground	H	M	H	M	M	M	H	M	M-H	L	H	L	H
Gaelic Football	H	M	H	M-H	M	M	H	M	M	L	M	L	H
Gymnastics													
a. Balance Beam	L	L	H	M-H	M-H	L	L	M	M	L	H	H	H
b. Floor Exercise	M	H	H	H	H	H	M	M	M	H	H	H	H
c. Horse	L	H	L	M-H	M-H	M-H	L	M	M	M	H	H	L
d. Horizontal Bar	L	H	L	H	H	M-H	L	M	M	H	L	H	L
e. Long Horse	L	M	M	L	M	M-H	L	M	M	L	L	L	L
f. Parallel Bars	L	H	M	H	M	L	L	L	M	H	H	H	H

(continued) FIGURE 34 / FITNESS BENEFITS OF SELECTED SPORTS

H—High, M—Medium, L—Low, M-H—Depends whether recreation (M) or Vigorous (H)

g. Rings	L	H	M	H	H	H	H	M	H	H	L
h. Trampoline	M-H	M	H	M	M	M	M	L	H	L	H
Hauling	H	M	H	M	M	M	H	M	M	H	H
Ice Boating	L	M-H	L-M	L	L	M	M	L	L	L	L
Ice Hockey	H	H	H	M-H	M	M	H	M	H	L	M
Jai Alai	M	H	H	M	H	H	H	M	M-H	L	H
Judo	H	H	H	H	H	H	H	H	H	M	H
Karate	H	H	H	H	H	H	H	H	H	M	H
Lacrosse	H	H	H	M	M	H	H	M	H	H	H
Lumberjack Activities	H	H	H	H	H	M	M	M	L-H	H	M
Motor Sports											
a. Boat	L	L	L	L	L	M	M	L	L	L	L
b. Car	L	L	L	M	M	M	M	L	L	L	L
c. Cycle	L	L	L	L	L	M	M	L	L	L	L
d. Plane	L	L	L	L	L	M	M	L	L	L	L
Parachute Jumping	L	L	L	L	L	L	L	L	L	L	L
Polo	M	M	L	M	L	M	M	M	M-H	H	L
Rodeo	M	H	H	H	M	M	M	M	M-H	H	H
Rugby	H	M-H	H	M	L	M	H	M	M	L	H
Scuba Diving	M	M	H	L	M	M	M	M	M	L	M
Soccer	H	L	L	M	M	M	M	M	H	M	H
Softball	L	M	M	M	L	M	L	M	L	L	H
Speedball	H	L	H	M	H	M	H	M	H	L	H
Surfing	L	L	M	L	L	L	M	L-M	L	L	M
Tennis	H-M	M	H	M	H	M	H	M	H	H	H

FIGURE 35 / FITNESS BENEFITS OF SELECTED SPORTS

H–High, M–Medium, L–Low, M-H–Depends whether recreation (M) or Vigorous (H)

Sport	C-R Endurance	Muscle Strength				Muscle Endurance				Flexibility			
		Arms	Legs	Abdomen	Back	Arms	Legs	Abdomen	Back	Shoulder	Hip	Elbow	Knee
Track & Field													
a. Sprints	M	M	H	M	M	M	M	M	M	L	H	L	H
b. Middle Distance	H	M	H	M	M	M	M	M	M	L	H	L	H
c. Long Distance	H	M	H	M	M	M	H	H	H	L	H	L	H
d. Marathon	H	M	H	M	M	H	H	H	H	L	H	L	H
e. Walking	H	M	H	M	M	M	H	H	H	L	H	L	H
f. 35 lb. weight throw	L	H	H	M	H	L	L	L	L	M-H	H	H	H
g. Shot Put	L	H	H	M	H	L	L	L	L	M-H	H	H	H
h. Pole Vault	L	H	H	H	H	M	M	M	M	H	H	H	H
i. Triple Jump	L	M	H	H	H	L	L	L	L	M	H	L	H
j. Hurdling	M	M	H	H	H	L	L	L	L	M	H	L	H
k. Discus Throw	L	H	H	M	H	L	L	L	L	M	H	H	H
l. Hammerthrow	L	H	H	M	H	L	L	L	L	H	H	H	H
m. High Jump	L	M	H	H	H	L	L	L	L	M	H	L	M
n. Javelin	L	H	H	M	H	L	L	L	L	M-H	H	H	H
o. Long Jump	L	M	H	H	H	L	L	L	L	M	H	L	H
Volleyball	M-H	M-H	M-H	M	M	M-H	M-H	M	M	M	M	H	M
Water Polo	M-H	H	M	L-M	L-M	H	H	M-H	M-H	M-H	M	H	M
Water Skiing	M-H	H	M-H	L-M	M	M-H	H	M-H	M-H	L	L	L	M
Weight Lifting	L	H	H	H	H	L-H	L-H	L-H	L-H	M	M	M	M
Wrestling	H	H	H	H	H	H	H	H	H	M-H	H	H	H

16

WHAT CAN EXERCISE EQUIPMENT DO FOR YOU?

ONE OF THE GREAT IRONIES OF MODERN-DAY AMERICA IS THE fact that exercise—the antithesis of sedentary, push-button living—is itself becoming automated. In the past, the evangelists of physical fitness heralded effort and sweat as the route to physical fitness. But now a new breed of self-proclaimed apostles is offering a host of machines and devices to those searching for physical vitality and good health.

The great majority of exercise equipment makers are reliable people with good consciences and good products. But it should come as a surprise to no one that a hundred-million-dollar-a-year industry that has grown over 300 percent in the past few years should attract some profiteers.

The idea is inviting—a new piece of exercise equipment that will help you lose weight, trim your waistline, and condition your heart, with absolutely no effort. An end to tiring exercise, jogging, and sweat.

Separating the good from the bad is a tough assignment. Dr. William Haskell, Ph.D., former program director for the President's Council on Physical Fitness and now assistant professor of preventive medicine at Stanford University, has made a statement worth repeating: "There seems to be an inverse relationship between the claims made and the actual effectiveness of the device." [1] The greater the claims, the poorer the device.

PASSIVE VERSUS ACTIVE EXERCISE

Exercise equipment works in one of two ways:

1 / active, in which the person works on the machines, and
2 / passive, in which the machine works on the individual (you permit yourself to be shaken, shocked, rolled, strapped, and girdled).

PASSIVE EQUIPMENT—NO-SWEAT EXERCISE

If you are using devices of the "passive" type, don't kid yourself into thinking they have much value. They may relax you and make you feel like a million bucks, but many authorities agree that such products make little if any contribution to fitness.[2] The American Medical Association's Committee on Exercise and Physical Fitness, for one, is skeptical: "Effortless exercise ... cannot benefit a person in any magical way." [3]

In short, if you are going to benefit from exercise, you must put effort into it. Do not be misled by health club claims that their machine is unique or doctor-approved. Passive exercise equipment cannot help you become fit, nor will it roll off the fat. The best advice on passive exercise is simple: If you don't have to work on the machine, forget it. Don't waste your money. Even the active devices aren't always what they are cracked up to be. Every exercise device must be judged with respect to its contributions to the five fitness components outlined earlier—circulo-respiratory endurance, body composition and weight, flexibility, muscle strength, and muscle endurance.

EVALUATING ACTIVE EQUIPMENT

Literally hundreds of exercise devices are on the market. *Consumer Guide®* here provides some guidelines for evaluating their specific fitness contributions. No one device will provide all the fitness benefits. Some may help you to increase circulatory fitness, others muscle strength, and still others muscle endurance. But none at the present time works on all five components. *Furthermore, it is not necessary to purchase any of these devices.* You can improve all the basic components of fitness without any equipment at all.

People use exercise devices for a variety of reasons:

1 / to get started on a fitness program
2 / to be able to exercise in the privacy of their home
3 / to exercise specific muscle groups
4 / to make it possible to exercise in any kind of weather
5 / to compensate for orthopedic problems

Consumer Guide® repeats its assertion, however, that for most people equipment is not necessary. For some people—those who are fascinated by such equipment or have a special reason to prefer using one or another device—equipment may be an important aid.

CIRCULO-RESPIRATORY ENDURANCE

To improve circulo-respiratory endurance, heart function, heart health, etc., a piece of equipment must permit endurance exercise of a sustained nature. The person exercising on the device must use the major muscle groups for twenty to thirty minutes. It must also permit exercise of sufficient vigor to get the heart rate into the target zone. The key here is to use your body muscles to get your pulse rate up to your target zone and to keep it there for more than just a few seconds; otherwise, the exercise is not of a continuous nature. Examples of those pieces of equipment which raise the heart rate for only a short period of time or which are not of a continuous endurance nature are weight training equipment and isokinetic devices. The only types that have been shown to hold the pulse rate at the target zone with continuous exercise are treadmills, stationary bicycles, rowing machines, and creeping devices.

BODY COMPOSITION

Two popular claims are made for the potential of exercise devices for altering body composition: a device may help you (1) lose weight or (2) redistribute fat.

As we've explained in earlier sections of this book, fat and extra weight accumulate as a result of inactivity and overeating. The only way to reverse the condition is to increase your activity level and decrease food intake. In short, the calorie outgo must exceed the calorie intake.

The rolling, massaging, and the like aren't going to do any good. Yet elaborate tables, couches, chairs, beds, cushions, belts, and small hand-held apparatuses at prices ranging from a few dollars to several hundred dollars are popular. They produce movement of your body, but you're not doing the moving! One report derides the extravagant claims of some equipment manufacturers: "It is incorrect to assert, as has been done, that forty-five minutes on a rocking table is equivalent, physically, to playing thirty-six holes of golf or riding ten miles at a canter. . . . All claims that vibrators are effective . . . promoting weight reduction are probably false and misleading." [4] Another researcher in this field found one device of dubious value. Dr. Arthur Steinhaus reported that the use of a vibrator belt for fifteen minutes a day for a year *might* produce a one- to one-and-a-half-pound weight loss, with no mobilization of body fat.[5]

Losing weight, like conditioning the heart and lungs, requires effort on your part, not a machine's. There is no other way, and the company that claims otherwise is pulling your leg. Once again, the only types of equipment that have been shown to help hold the pulse at the target zone with continuous exercise (and thus provide weight and fat-control benefits) are treadmills, stationary bicycles, and rowing machines.

Closely allied with loss of weight (and body fat) is change in muscle mass. Exercise with devices that improve muscle strength and endurance may affect body composition by increasing muscle mass. Those contributing to muscle strength and endurance (see below) will increase the amount of lean body tissue and change body composition.

MUSCLE STRENGTH

If a device is advertised as improving muscle strength, it should cause the muscles to be exerted to at least two thirds of maximum effort. For example, if you can lift a maximum of one hundred pounds over your head, a lifting exercise to improve arm and shoulder strength would have to require you to lift sixty-seven pounds above your head several times every other day.

Isometric (no movement), isotonic (movement), or isokinetic (combination of isometric and isotonic) exercises may be used. Strength improvement by the isometric method involves maximal contraction of the muscle for five seconds, five to ten times or more a day. For weight-training exercises (isotonic), three sets of six repetitions maximum is required to improve muscle strength for a particular muscle group. The weight must be heavy enough so that no more than ten repetitions of an exercise can be done without tiring. For strength to be improved through isokinetic exercise, it is necessary to follow the regimen outlined for you by the manufacturer.

Devices currently available for improving muscle strength include standard barbells and dumbbells, multiple-station gyms, heavy-springed devices, and isokinetic devices (such as Exer-Genie, Apollo, Mini-Gym, Exer-Gym). Any of these can be effective provided it is used properly and often enough.

MUSCLE ENDURANCE

If a device is to improve muscle endurance, it must exercise the muscle to the point of fatigue—at which point continued exertion is practically impossible. If the work load is too great, however, so that you must stop after only a few contractions, strength rather than endurance is being developed. You should be able to do at least fifteen to thirty repetitions before having to stop.

Weight training is a good example of exercise to build muscle endurance. Most exercise equipment designed to increase muscle strength (with the exception of isometric devices) can also be used to improve muscle endurance. For endurance training, the emphasis is placed on repeating the exercise a considerable number of times with a lighter weight or lighter resistance than in strength-building.

FLEXIBILITY

A device that claims to increase flexibility should allow the muscles, tendons, and ligaments to go through their full range of motion. There should be a complete contraction and extension of these tissues. Flexibility requires stretching movements. An isometric exercise will not improve flexibility.

Very few devices on the market today claim to improve flexibility, yet it should be considered. Lack of flexibility will leave you more prone to injury. Exercise can be quite effective; most muscle strength and endurance exercises (except for isometrics) can be used to improve flexibility provided they are done properly.

NEBULOUS CLAIMS TO HOOK THE UNWARY

"Our device improves muscle tone." This is a famous and oft-used expression in the advertising of many exercise equipment companies. Conflicting evidence and research have been cited as to whether muscle tone is improved with exercise or not. In fact, muscle tone is a controversial term in itself.

Exactly what is muscle tone? It is the state of contraction of a muscle even while you are at rest. The degree of contraction is dependent upon the response of the muscle to the nervous system. The tone will vary depending upon the stimulation received from the nervous system whether you are lying down or standing up. Manufacturers would be hard put to prove that their device improves muscle tone. It is not known whether exercise itself, let alone mechanical exercise, has an effect on muscle tone: "There is no reason to believe that the use of a vibratory abdominal belt, vibratory bed, pillow, or other device will 'tone up' muscles so as to reduce girth." [6]

Personal testimonials by famous people are another questionable technique used to promote exercise devices. Sometimes a coincidence is used to promote a product dishonestly. For example, if an entire football team of a university used a particular exercise device in training and then won a championship that year, the manufacturer might claim the product deserved the credit.

Another popular advertising approach that should be regarded with suspicion is the type that announces that using a piece of equipment for three to six minutes a day will provide all the benefits of swimming a mile or jogging two miles. Unless using the equipment increases the pulse to a rate equivalent to that achieved by swimming or jogging itself, and keeps it there as long as the exercise would, claims to the effect that the product is equally useful are false. In addition, the device must burn as many calories as the exercise and stress the same muscle groups to work off fat or to do the same amount of work in order to support the claims made for it.

"Spot reducing" is another favorite advertising term. It implies that it is possible to reduce the amount of fat at a particular part of the body by performing certain exercises. That's physiological hogwash. We've already explained that fat is stored in fat cells throughout the body and that when energy is needed, it is released from all over the body.

Unfortunately, useless and falsely advertised exercise equipment has resulted in a certain skepticism toward all such devices, even some that may really help you. Often the products are fine, but the claims are excessive and even sometimes downright false. If you are fully aware of the limitations and the potential benefits, you are more likely to be a satisfied customer.

EVALUATING EXERCISE EQUIPMENT

Three exercise physiologists were contacted by *Consumer Guide*® to make comments about various types of equipment available. They are Dr. William Day, Ph.D., Director of New England Cardiovascular Health Institute, Cambridge, MA; Dr. Michael Pollock, Ph.D., Director of Research, Institute for Aerobic Research, Dallas, TX; and Dr. William Zuti, Ph.D., Assistant Professor, Department of Health, Physical Education, and Recreation, Kansas State University, Manhattan, Kansas.

Prior to making their evaluations, each expert was asked to offer some general comments about exercise equipment.

Dr. Day: "My basic concern about physical fitness equipment is whether people will use the equipment for any extended period of time. My feeling is that if people are really sincere in their attempt to become fit, then it's possible for them to achieve those goals without equipment. A well-motivated person might find treadmills and bicycles helpful in inclement weather or if they have some medical condition that requires a more controlled workout."

Dr. Pollock: "Exercise equipment can be useful in an exercise program, but the equipment is not mandatory or even necessary. Many times you can accomplish the same thing without equipment. The advantage of equipment is that it can be used indoors. If you want to develop strength, then weights and weight training equipment might be useful."

Dr. Zuti: "Exercise equipment is not a necessity for fitness. But people like to use equipment for motivational purposes, which is okay, provided they use them. Some equipment is good, such as treadmills, while others are out-and-out quackery."

EVALUATION OF PASSIVE EQUIPMENT

Whirlpool Baths—These may include portable or self-contained units, the purpose of which is to direct water forcefully at your body. The moving water is to provide a massage; some are gentle and some are not so gentle.

According to the Experts: "Whirlpool baths may be helpful in bringing temporary relief to minor aches and pains due to overexertion. But they are of no real fitness value."

Consumer Guide® Rating: Whirlpool baths are not recommended for fitness improvement.

Belt Vibrators—The belt vibrator is simply a motorized belt that is supposed to shake or vibrate the fat off your body.

According to the Experts: "Belt vibrators are not effective in improving fitness. There is absolutely no evidence to support the contention that fat can be rolled, shaken, or vibrated off the body. Vibrators are nice for relaxing, but they do not contribute one iota to fitness. They are a waste of money. They don't burn calories, and they don't redistribute or remove fat. They may be dangerous for people with varicose veins."

Consumer Guide® Rating: Belt vibrators are not recommended.

Roller Machines—These are the devices which have a series of rollers that are supposed to massage the fat off specific areas of the body.

According to the Experts: "A complete waste of money. There is no way any kind of external massage, rolling, or bumping will cause fat to be removed. Roller machines don't burn calories. In fact, they may be dangerous for people with varicose veins or other circulatory disorders."

Consumer Guide® Rating: Roller machines are not recommended.

EVALUATION OF ACTIVE EQUIPMENT

Treadmills—These are devices on which you walk. They usually have a heavy-gauge steel frame which supports a belt that moves as you walk. Since a treadmill is a type of conveyor belt, you simple walk in place. Two basic types of treadmills are available—motorized and nonmotorized. The motorized type has a motor which moves the belt, forcing you to walk or run on the belt at a selected speed. The incline of the treadmill can also be adjusted on many motorized treadmills in order to simulate walking or running uphill. Consequently, the exercise becomes more difficult.

According to the Experts: "Motor-driven treadmills are excellent pieces of equipment for cardiovascular improvement. They are especially good for use in inclement weather. They are expensive, however, and storage is difficult. Also, with one of the larger models adequate head room can be a problem. For some people, these machines are boring."

Consumer Guide® Rating: Although an excellent piece of equipment, a motorized treadmill is quite expensive.

The nonmotorized treadmills operate on a different principle. When you walk or run, your feet cause the belt to move. A flywheel keeps the treadmill belt moving at an even speed.

According to the Experts: "Nonmotorized treadmills are much less expensive than the motor-driven ones. They are satisfactory for walking, but they are not recommended for running because of foot irritation."

Consumer Guide® Rating: The nonmotorized treadmill is a good product for people who have difficulty getting outdoors and must confine their fitness efforts to walking.

Stationary Bicycles—Stationary bicycles are exactly what their name implies—bicycles which remain stationary as you pedal. They come in all sizes, shapes, and models. Some are motorized and others nonmotorized. Nonmotorized bikes look like any other bicycle except the back wheel is missing. The chain from the pedal sprocket goes to the front wheel, which turns when you pedal. Most bikes have a knob which allows you to adjust pedal resistance by increasing or decreasing the pressure of the brake shoes on the front wheel.

According to the Experts: "Nonmotorized bicycles are excellent pieces of equipment for cardiovascular improvement. They are good for cardiac patients who need a precise measurement of the amount of work they've done, but they can be boring and a loss of leg flexibility can occur. Be sure the bicycle has a means of telling you the speed and resistance on the wheel."

Consumer Guide® Rating: The nonmotorized stationary bicycle is an excellent product for improvement of cardio-respiratory fitness.

The motorized bicycle works on a different principle. Here

the motor causes the pedals to turn. Consequently, your legs are not required to do the work. The motor also causes the bike's handlebar to move forward and backward and the seat to move up and down. As a result, there is a great deal of body motion. But the motion is motor-induced, not self-induced.

According to the Experts: "Motorized bicycles are probably overrated. While a cardiovascular workout can be elicited by working against the machine, little benefit is derived if you let the machine do the work for you. This type of bicycle can be cumbersome and uncomfortable. It is difficult to measure work done. It can also be dangerous to the uninitiated. You can get the same benefit from the nonmotorized bicycle at one fifth of the cost."

Consumer Guide® Rating: The motorized stationary bicycle is not recommended.

Rowing Machines—A rowing machine is a device which is designed to simulate the body action of rowing a boat. The rowing machine has a seat which moves along a steel frame as you exercise by moving the oars. As you pull back on the oars the seat moves, and as you release the oars forward the seat moves again. Consequently, the upper body and legs get some exercise.

According to the Experts: "A moderately expensive device that is good for cardiovascular fitness and weight control, the rowing machine can be strenuous and may not be recommended for people with heart disease problems. The problem is that the extensive use of the upper body may cause blood pressure to rise excessively."

Consumer Guide® Rating: Although the rowing machine is recommended as a good cardiovascular product for most people, it is not for use by people with high blood pressure or victims of cardiovascular disease.

Creeping Devices—A creeping device is a compact unit with tracks on which two hand carriages and two knee carriages slide back and forth. The carriages are linked together so that all four move in unison. To exercise, you place your hands on the hand carriages and your knees on the knee carriages and move them back and forth as though you were creeping. It was originally designed to help children and adults improve coordination, but more recently a manufacturer has claimed it can improve cardio-respiratory fitness.

According to the Experts: "Probably can be used effectively to burn calories and stimulate the cardiovascular system. The basic problem with the creeping device is that it is extremely boring and most people will not stick with it."

Consumer Guide® Rating: Creeping devices receive a good rating, but their application is quite limited.

Isokinetic Devices—According to the Experts: "These products are designed primarily for muscle strength and muscle endurance. They are not good cardiovascular exercisers. They have an advantage over weight training in that you do not have to lift a dead weight. One major disadvantage is that since the poundages on the cylinder are estimates, people become frustrated in that they don't know how much work they're doing."

Consumer Guide® Rating: Recommended for the development of strength only, isokinetic devices receive a poor rating as overall fitness products.

Weight Training and Mini-Gyms—According to the Experts: "These are good for the development of muscle strength and muscle endurance, but they are not really necessary for the average adult. Most people can build enough strength with a good calisthenics program. May be helpful to the person who wants to work on some muscle strength deficiencies or improve the strength of their sports game. Young athletes will be able to use them to good advantage for strength development."

Consumer Guide® Rating: These products are recommended for strength development only; they receive a poor rating as overall fitness products.

Exercise Wheel—The exercise wheel is a product which looks like the wheel of a small wagon or a lawn mower with a dowel sticking out both sides. To exercise with the product you get into a creeping position resting on your knees and placing your hands on the dowels of the wheel. Then you extend your body as far out as possible by pushing the wheel on the ground. Once extended as far as possible, you are to return to the starting position. Repeated several times, the exercise is supposed to trim your waistline.

According to the Experts: "A real gimmick item, the exercise wheel offers few advantages, if any. It is a device which places you in an uncomfortable position, and can possibly be harmful to a person's lower back."

Consumer Guide® Rating: The exercise wheel is not recommended.

Rubber Stretchers—The rubber stretchers are highly elastic pieces of rubber with loops at the ends for easier gripping and holding. To use the product you are to grip the loops and then pull your arms apart as far as possible. Or you can place your foot in one loop and then pull up with the opposite arm.

According to the Experts: "A rubber stretcher can develop strength of specific muscles. Of questionable value to adults who are interested in maintaining good health, it doesn't allow any leeway for changes in strength. You may be a very weak person who is unable to move it. On the other hand, you may be quite strong and find the resistance too low."

Consumer Guide® Rating: Rubber stretchers are not recommended.

Chest Pulls—Chest pulls operate on the same principle as the rubber stretchers. The chest pulls are usually made up of two detachable handles with one to five rubber or steel-spring cables between. The object of the chest pull is to pull the handles apart. How far you can pull them depends upon your strength. The detachable handles permit you to have one to five cables. This allows you to make adjustments depending upon your strength.

According to the Experts: "The spring chest pull can help develop muscle strength in specific muscles, particularly the arms, shoulders, and the chest. It certainly should not be used by persons with cardiac conditions. As with the rubber stretcher, it is very difficult to know how much work is being done, and little leeway is made for changes in strength—although springs may be added or removed. When the springs are stretched they can trap the user's skin and cause a nasty pinch when released."

Consumer Guide® Rating: Chest pulls are not recommended.

Body Trimmers—Body trimmers were the rage during 1975 and 1976. They are simply pulley and rope systems, which you attach to a wall, door, etc. You then lie flat on the floor with your feet and hands attached to the ropes. As you move your leg downward, your arm will be pulled forward and vice versa.

According to the Experts: "Body trimmers use one set of muscles to work against the other set. If they were properly used and an individual could regulate the resistance, he or she might derive some benefit. A person is better off to stick with calisthenics than to waste his money on such a gimmick."

Consumer Guide® Rating: Body trimmers are not recommended.

Isometric Exercisers—Isometric exercisers cover a wide range of products. They may involve exerting against a rope, or they may have you pulling on a cord or pushing one cylinder inside another that has been programmed for a certain amount of resistance.

According to the Experts: "Isometric exercisers can produce muscle strength if used properly, but they should not be used by cardiac patients or by people with high blood pressure. The very limited benefits can be duplicated by performing such exercises as pushing against door jambs, etc."

Consumer Guide® Rating: Isometric products receive a poor rating.

Jump Rope—Jump ropes come in all shapes and sizes. Some are cotton, others are nylon, polyethylene, or hemp. Some are autographed, others are not. Some have handles or weighted ends, others do not. Some are packaged with books, others have small pamphlets to accompany them. In other words, you can almost call your own shots in picking a rope.

According to the Experts: "A jump rope is an excellent piece of exercise equipment if used regularly. The big danger is that some people believe that only a few minutes of rope skipping will produce significant changes. Rope skipping is not magical. To derive cardiovascular benefit you must exercise at a target rate of 70 to 85 percent of maximum. Some people may get bored with the scenery. There is no need to purchase a special rope. Sash cord or heavy wash line will do."

Consumer Guide® Rating: An excellent piece of equipment. But remember: The oft-made claim that ten minutes of rope skipping is equivalent to thirty minutes of jogging is not accurate. That statement is based on one study reported in 1968.* A careful analysis of the study, however, reveals some serious shortcomings. One is that the people skipping rope exercised at a much harder rate than those who jogged. The test used to measure fitness progress was based on heart rate recovery—hardly an adequate test for measuring fitness improvement.

---

* J. A. Baker, "Comparison of Rope Skipping and Jogging as Methods of Improving Cardiovascular Efficiency of College Men," *Research Quarterly*, May, 1968, p. 240.

17

THE SWEAT, STEAM, SAUNA ROUTE TO NOWHERE

FOR YEARS SWEATING HAS BEEN EQUATED WITH WEIGHT LOSS, getting fit, and ridding the body of waste. Nothing could be farther from the truth. Here is another subject surrounded with misinformation, half-truths, and out-and-out deceit.

SWEAT: YOUR INTERNAL THERMOSTAT

The human body can be compared to an engine with a thermostat, except that the human thermostat cannot be turned off. The body produces heat in many ways—cell activity, muscular activity, digestion of food, and production of hormones, for example. It also picks up heat from the sun or from the rays of the sun bouncing off sand or snow.

Whatever the source, the body must protect itself from accumulating too much heat. Under normal conditions heat is lost in a number of ways—through the skin, through sweat, through the lungs, and through waste.

During exercise, the situation changes; then sweat be-

272

comes a most important key to keeping the body cool. For sweat to produce a loss of heat, it must evaporate (sweat that is wiped away or permitted to run off the body has no cooling function). As sweat evaporates, it cools the blood close to the surface of the skin. That blood returns to the body's inner core tissues. At the same time, the interior blood is carrying heat from the deeper tissues toward the skin, where the heat can be lost to the environment. Circulation is speeded up during exercise, which makes the heat exchange more efficient.

In an atmosphere of low humidity, sweat will evaporate very quickly into the dry air. Likewise, when a breeze is blowing, the currents will aid evaporation. But if the humidity is high (which means the air is saturated with water), sweat cannot be taken up by the air, and the water simply drips off the body. The blood near the skin surface is not cooled, the temperature of the core tissue is not lowered, and the body temperature continues to rise.

Heat exhaustion is the body's reaction to a sustained period of inhibition of sweat evaporation. The blood rushes quickly to the body surface in an effort to carry the core heat to the skin where sweat evaporation can disperse it. As the blood flows to the surface capillaries, the blood pressure drops. At the same time, blood volume is reduced because some of the liquid does pass into the skin cells and evaporate as sweat. As the heart becomes less able to maintain blood pressure, there is a slowdown in circulation. The core heat no longer escapes the body, and heat exhaustion occurs.

The general signs of heat exhaustion are profuse sweating, moist skin, and rapid pulse. The person is usually very uncomfortable and gasps for breath. Collapse and loss of consciousness may follow. The victim needs fluids and rest; recovery is usually rapid.

Dehydration exhaustion occurs when a person does not take in enough water while exercising. During very heavy exercise, when sweating very hard, the average person may lose eight quarts of water in ninety minutes. Even in moderate exercise, water loss is around three quarts in ninety minutes, which is practically impossible to replenish in ninety minutes. Consequently, there's a decrease in blood volume. A stimulus is sent to the hypothalamus which in turn signals the release of a hormone to slow down the production of urine so that water is conserved.

If profuse sweating continues and the fluid lost is not replaced, *heat stroke* develops. This is a medical emergency, and a doctor must be called immediately. Heat stroke is characterized by a rising temperature and very dry skin. Unless the temperature is promptly reduced, permanent damage to the cells of the brain will occur—and very probably death.

How does heat stroke develop? It starts with a rise in skin temperature, followed by sweating and expansion of the blood vessels (vasodilation). As the temperature continues to rise, further vasodilation and sweating take place. Soon the point is reached where sweating efficiency decreases. When that happens, the blood is no longer cooled adequately, the core temperature rises, sweating ceases altogether, and heat stroke occurs.[1]

The loss of water is only part of the problem. Under heavy sweating the body also loses many electrolytes (sodium, chloride, and potassium). A prolonged loss of electrolytes and water may cause nausea, diarrhea, and fatigue, and may impair kidney functioning to the point where kidney tissue damage occurs.[2]

THE SWEATY PATH TO FITNESS?

Misconceptions about the relationship of sweating to weight loss and fitness have led to some controversial practices. *Consumer Guide*® has selected the most well known of these practices for discussion.

RUBBERIZED (NONPOROUS) AND HEAVY SWEATSUITS

Nonporous sweatsuits and extremely heavy exercise clothing enclose the body in a hot environment that can cause body temperature to rise to dangerous levels.[3] The surface of the skin is deprived of exposure to the air. The suit traps the heat given off by the body, and sweat does not evaporate. As a result, body temperature starts to climb very rapidly and one of the conditions previously described—heat exhaustion, dehydration exhaustion, or heat stroke—can occur.

Why do people wear these nonporous suits? Most users believe it is a quick way to lose weight; they can be five pounds lighter after the workout. Unfortunately, this is not correct. After a good workout and sweating profusely, you may find that you have lost three to five pounds or even more, but that weight loss is only water (not fat) and it is only temporary. As soon as you drink liquid you will start to put the weight back on.

Dr. Laurence E. Morehouse, Ph.D., explains that excessive sweating is not desirable. "If a disproportionate share of that energy is used to secrete sweat, then there isn't enough left for your other bodily functions. The amount of work you can do lessens when sweat glands use energy. When exhausted, they stop secreting and you are in peril of a heat stroke." [4]

Morehouse describes another problem of overheating: the drain on the cardiovascular system. When the skin gets hot, vessels near the skin surface open and a large part of your blood supply rushes to these surface capillaries. "This deprives the muscles of the blood they need. The heart tries to make up for the loss by pumping harder. The load becomes so great that if it's maintained for a prolonged period you could collapse, and conceivably die." [5] Morehouse concludes firmly that induced sweating is dangerous.

"In exercise, you can control the pumping of your heart simply by stopping what you are doing. But when you overload your heart by overheating your body [such as with rubberized sweatsuits], there's no way you can stop the process except by jumping into some ice water." [6]

Consumer Guide® cautions against the use of rubberized or extremely heavy sweatsuits. They do not make a contribution to fitness. Worse, they prevent the body from cooling itself, and the consequences can be disastrous. This is true even if the suits cover only one part of the anatomy. Heavy sweatsuits are especially hazardous in warm climates, but even in cool climates they should be used judiciously. Lightweight jogging suits are acceptable provided they are made of a porous material.

STEAMROOMS

Steamrooms are popular attractions in many health clubs. The temperature in a steamroom is held at 110° to 130° Fahrenheit, with humidity also very high. A person who sits in the steamroom will, of course, sweat profusely. Because of the very high humidity, the sweat cannot evaporate and cannot have a cooling effect on the body. As a result, body temperatures can rise to dangerous levels. Doctors Clayton R. Myers, Ph.D., Lawrence Golding, Ph.D., and Wayne Sinning, Ph.D., write in their book, "There is growing concern among physicians that ... steam baths may be detrimental to health. Heat stress is not tolerated well by most middle-aged people. Heat exposure can lead to heat exhaustion. The dangers of heat exposure are increased if an individual enters the bath after exercise, when the body is trying to reduce its temperature." [7]

Consumer Guide® regards steamrooms as detrimental to health. The steam bath makes no contribution to fitness.

SAUNA

The sauna concept is similar to that of the steamroom and nonporous sweatsuits, with one important difference. In the sauna, the temperature is high *but the humidity is kept low.* The low-humidity air is better able to pick up sweat from the surface of the skin. Consequently, the body is better able to maintain proper temperature.

Many claims have been made for the sauna. The great majority of these claims, however, have appeared in popular magazines and newspapers, in articles thin in research and high in personal testimonials. Claims have also been made, of course, by sauna manufacturers and representatives. Some may be legitimate, others exaggerated or misleading, and still others false. *Consumer Guide®* has selected twelve of the sauna's purported benefits for evaluation.

1. The sauna will raise body temperature. Doctors Jeddi Hansen, M.D., Matti Karvonen, M.D., and Pekka Piironen confirm this statement.[8] The degree of increase will depend upon the length of time in the sauna, air temperature, humidity, and body position. However, the desirability of the higher body temperature is unclear.

2. The sauna will relax muscles and tranquilize the nervous system. This is one of the most frequently heard comments on the sauna. People say they feel more relaxed or less tense after taking a sauna. There may be good reason for this feeling. Dr. Herbert deVries, Ph.D., measured with electromyographic instruments the electrical activity in the musculature of sixteen subjects as they took a sauna bath. He determined that the sauna brings about a significant decrease in neuromuscular activity. Heart rate, systolic and diastolic blood pressures were all lower after the sauna. Furthermore, the magnitude of the effect was approximately proportional to the activity level that existed prior to the sauna. Thus the greatest benefits are derived by those who are in need of a tranquilizing effect. Evidence suggested the following explanation:

1 / Increased body temperature decreases gamma motor nerve activity.

2 / Decreased innervation of the muscle fibers results in less proprioceptive input.

3 / The decrease in proprioceptive input results in decreased reflex alpha innervation and decreased resting neuromuscular activity.

The investigators concluded that sauna bath procedures can bring about a significant decrease in the activity of the neuromuscular system.[9]

One criticism of deVries' study was that all sixteen subjects were patients in a physical rehabilitation center and that no similar results have been obtained with other subjects.

Work conducted by Dr. Marliese Lehtments, M.D., reported that subjects experienced a relief from nervous tension and had more favorable attitudes after being in the sauna.[10]

3. The sauna relieves muscle aches and pains. Muscle aches and pains are very difficult ailments to pinpoint. If they are due to muscular or nervous tension, it is conceivable that the sauna may relax the muscles or tranquilize the nervous system, thereby relieving the aches and pains. Not enough research has been done to confirm or discount this contention.

4. The sauna leads to more restful sleep. Here again, evidence is lacking, but common sense suggests this statement may be justified. If the sauna relieves muscle tension and tranquilizes the nervous system, or if people feel better after the sauna, it may indeed help set the stage for more restful sleep.

5. A sauna bath eliminates body poisons. The sauna enthusiasts may be on dangerous ground here. You sweat to keep your cool. Sweating causes a tremendous loss of water and electrolytes, which can have a harmful effect on the body, as we've already explained.

On the other hand, the sauna may be of value to chronic dialysis patients. A report in *Medical World News* describes a program at Peter Bent Brigham Hospital in Boston, in which patients with kidney failure were put on sauna therapy for half an hour every day. Tests indicated that urea nitrogen, a waste product usually eliminated from the body in the urine but which remains in the blood when the kidneys do not operate properly, was secreted in the sweat of the patients in concentrations ten times that of control groups.[11] The sauna also remarkably reduced the itching sensation that often accompanies chronic uremia; in six patients, the itching eventually disappeared entirely. The researchers noted that there were no abnormal side effects (some subjects had more than 250 sauna baths).

6. *The sauna improves circulation.* Are the sauna enthusiasts here referring to heart action, cardiac output, blood pressure, peripheral circulation, or what? Dr. M. L. Lehtments observes that findings about blood pressure readings in the sauna have not always been the same. Individual responses and experimental conditions have varied extensively, with thirteen studies or observers noting an increase in systolic blood pressure when taking the sauna and six reporting a decrease.[12] The complexity and individuality of factors regulating blood pressures are probably the main reasons for the inconsistencies.

Richard C. Warner summarized his investigation of the effects of sauna on improved circulation: "Investigators corroborate that subcutaneous circulation does increase. Temporarily, there is a general improvement in circulation which could affect the limb extremities. No known experiments have studied the long-term improvement in circulation. Functional circulatory disorders respond well to the cardiovascular effect of sauna bathing."[13]

7. Sauna bathing causes a loss of weight. We've already stated that the only way to lose weight is to burn off more calories than you take in. Sitting in a hot sauna does not burn significant numbers of calories. Whatever weight is lost in a hot environment is a loss of water and not fat tissue. Yes, you may be three pounds lighter after a sauna bath, but you will gain it back almost as soon as you eat or drink.[14]

8. Sauna clears up skin ailments and blemishes. Dr. Harry Johnson, M.D., of the Life Extension Institute reports that research does not support the claim that sauna baths correct acne, eczema, or other skin conditions.[15] The body is neither detoxified nor cleansed by excessive perspiration.

9. Sauna baths help to cure and prevent colds. The review by Richard Warner states, "There is no medical evidence to prove that sauna shortens or prevents the common cold. Sauna is contraindicated for those with colds." [16]

10. Sauna increases fitness. In 1964 Dr. Bengt Saltin, Ph.D., reported a study in which four subjects were dehydrated in a sauna. They were then exercised on a bicycle ergometer at various levels of muscular work up to their individual maximum. The investigator measured body weight, oxygen uptake, heart rate, plasma volume, hemoglobin concentration and blood, hematocrit, and cardiac output. He found that the decrease in body weight was accompanied by a reduction in plasma volume of up to 25 percent. After the sauna bath and submaximal exercise, there was a decrease in stroke volume and an associated increase in heart rate, so that the cardiac output remained almost the same. Dehydration produced no significant changes in oxygen uptake, cardiac output, or stroke volume when combined with maximal exercise. Further measurements suggested that exposure to the sauna resulted in decreased ability to perform maximum work.[17]

Dr. Matti Karvonen, M.D., Ph.D., conducted a series of experiments in which he found that there was a decrease in muscular strength of 7 percent one hour after exposure to the sauna. Further investigation did not reveal appreciable strength changes. Karvonen concluded that the sauna probably doesn't affect strength—negatively or positively.[18]

11. The sauna aids in curing arthritis and bursitis. In his review of sauna studies, Richard Warner concluded, "There is no evidence that arthritis and/or bursitis might be alleviated by sauna. . . . It is possible that with relaxation, soft tissues become more tranquil, thus reducing aches in muscles and joints temporarily." [19]

12. Sauna benefits all people. The Federal Trade Commission warns that sauna baths may imperil the health of the elderly or sick.[20]

Consumer Guide® Rating: The sauna does not improve anyone's fitness level. It is not to be regarded as a means to achieve physical fitness. It may, however, make a contribution to relaxation and "feeling good," two important health objectives.

If you choose to use the sauna to help you relax and feel better, *Consumer Guide*® recommends these guidelines:

1 / The temperature should not be higher than 185° Fahrenheit and the humidity should be kept low— about 10 percent.

2 / Wear as little clothing as possible. Stark naked is best—no towel, no jewelry, watch, or eyeglasses.

3 / Beginners should spend no more than eight to ten minutes in the sauna and should be sure there is another person in attendance. Maximum time for the veteran sauna user is fifteen minutes.

4 / Never go into a sauna with a full stomach. Wait at least an hour—two hours are better—after a heavy meal.

5 / Never use a sauna when you are under the influence of alcohol or narcotics, or when you've taken antihistamines, tranquilizers, vasoconstrictors, vasodilators, stimulants, or hypnotics.

6 / Elderly people and those who suffer from diabetes, heart disease, or high blood pressure should probably avoid saunas altogether.[21]

SAUNA SHORTS AND BELTS (INFLATABLE OUTFITS)

A few years ago inflatable outfits were the rage. Sweat belts, girdles, or rubberized Bermuda shorts promised to take off ten inches around the waist in two weeks without dieting.

Many people were convinced these garments worked. They measured their waist and hips, donned the inflatable outfit, did the prescribed exercises, took off the inflatable outfit after several minutes or hours, and then remeasured themselves. Lo and behold, they were slimmer—for a time. If they had measured their hips a few hours later, they'd have found they were back to their old size. Why?

Here's what happened: The sauna shorts generated intense heat, and the cells directly underneath the shorts lost a great deal of water. So the cells did "shrink" in size, and the result was a loss in inches. But again there was no real loss of tissue—only water. As the wearer took in food or liquids, the cells regained the water they had lost and the wearer "regained" the inches. Some wearers, of course, countered that they simply wouldn't drink anything. To this argument one writer responds that it may be possible to prolong the effect of the shorts by limiting food and drink for a time, but the body eventually demands fluids (you can't go without water more than seventy-two hours). The liquid will soon be restored to the cells.[22]

In short, the theory of inches lost by inflatable outfits is pure bunk. Research supports this stand. Chris MacIntyre reported on two studies she and an associate conducted in which they compared weight and measurements of several groups of people—some wearing inflatable apparatus, some wearing none, and some on a low-calorie diet. All performed comparable exercise routines. The only significant difference among groups after the exercise and diet regimens was a weight loss among those who had dieted. "Our conclusion from all this research: Inches can be lost using an inflatable apparatus only if the user is on a 900- to 1,000-calorie-per-day diet." [23]

Dr. Clayton Myers, Ph.D., reached similar conclusions: "There is no evidence that [sauna belts] will contribute to any fat reduction. A recent Federal Trade Commission decision has restricted advertising these devices since the evidence in support of these claims was insufficient." [24]

For the most part, the devices are not dangerous. It is conceivable that a person with high blood pressure, coronary artery disease, or extreme obesity may have some problems with them. The outfits can cause excessive constriction of the blood vessels and for this reason can be dangerous.

One interesting legal case was brought against a sauna belt company. In October, 1972, the U.S. Postal Service won a suit against Sauna Belt Incorporated, a major promoter of a quick waistline-reduction program. According to the judge, the sauna belt program was "not a marvel of ease as claimed by advertising, but involved considerable effort, exertion, and discomfort to a considerable number of people engaging in it." [25]

Consumer Guide® Rating: The sauna belt is pure hokum. No one should spend money on such a piece of equipment.

18

PASSIVE EXERCISE: HERE'S THE RUB

IN THIS SEDENTARY AGE OF OVERWEIGHT, WE WOULD ALL like to find an "effortless" means of weight control and physical fitness. In this chapter, we'll look at a few approaches that ask very little of you.

YOUR FAT CELLS

The number of fat cells in your body is determined early in life, perhaps even before birth.[1] Some researchers believe the number of such cells may increase during the first three years and others suggest the number may not stabilize until adolescence. In adulthood, it is the *size* and not the number of fat cells that increases. When you are young and physically active, the fat cells are relatively low in fat content. But as you become more sedentary and burn off fewer calories, your cells fill up with fat--a special form of fat called triglyceride. (The fat in a fat cell is approximately 95-percent triglyceride.) [2]

Exactly how the fat gets into the fat cells has not been finally determined, but it is believed that the number of fat cells, the rate of fat circulation, enzyme action, and nervous and hormonal factors all play a role in depositing fat in the body.[3] A blood vessel and nerve are attached to each fat cell or group of fat cells; the nervous system can trigger the release of fat, which the circulatory system then distributes.

The exact way in which the fat gets out of the cell is another unsettled issue, but here again research points out a combination of factors, including the circulatory, nervous, endocrine, and muscular systems.[4] A key element appears to be hormonal action.

Insulin and adrenalin are thought to play critical roles in fat synthesis (insulin) and fat dissolving (adrenalin). Insulin tends to increase appetite because it reduces blood glucose levels. Adrenalin increases the blood glucose levels and encourages fat mobilization.[5] Another hormone, a growth hormone, has the main metabolic function of increasing the rate of breaking down fat.[6] Other research suggests that testosterone and corticoids also play an important role in fat deposition and removal.[7]

Dr. Jerome Knittle, M.D., sums it up: "Hormonal actions can markedly affect adipose-cell size by virtue of their effect on metabolism and cellular proliferation." [8]

In short, getting fat into and out of cells is the function of a complicated biochemical mechanism that involves almost every body system—nervous, circulatory, endocrine, digestive, muscular, etc.

MASSAGE

Misconceptions about massage abound. Far too often, the teaching of massage has been done by lay people who do not know much about physiology and are misled regarding the potential contribution of massage.

First, a definition: "Massage is defined as a systematic manipulation of soft tissue of the body for therapeutic purposes." [9] According to Dr. Miland E. Knapp, M.D., the effects of massage may be classified as "reflex" and "mechanical." [10] Reflex refers to the pleasurable sensations felt with massage, resulting in relaxed muscles and reduction of mental tension. Mechanical effects include improving return flow circulation of blood and lymph, stretching adhesions between muscle fibers, and mobilizing accumulations of fluid. Dr. Knapp acknowledges a long list of benefits of massage:

> Massage is useful in any condition requiring relief of pain, reduction of swelling or mobilization of contracted tissues. Probably the most important single indication of its use is the swelling and induration which often follow trauma. At certain stages of recovery, massage may be helpful in treating fractures, dislocations, sprains, strains, bruises and other injuries to tendons, nerves, and joints. It may benefit patients with arthritis, peri-arthritis, bursitis, neuritis, fibrositis, low back pain, cerebral palsy, multiple sclerosis, or paralytic conditions such as hemiplegia, paraplegia, and quadriplegia.[11]

Dr. Knapp cautions that people who have infections, malignancies, and skin diseases or disorders should not have massage and that massage does not develop muscle strength.

Unfortunately, many people are unaware of these valid functions of massage and believe that it is a means of getting rid of fat. One writer states, "This breaks down the fat so that it can be carried away by the bloodstream." [12] No documentation was given for this interpretation because there is none.

Massage may be great for relieving tension, but it is useless as a means of improving circulo-respiratory endurance, muscle strength, muscle endurance, and body composition. It may enhance flexibility if the lack of flexibility is due to muscle tension; massage can help to relieve the tension and, therefore, allow the muscle or muscle group to relax so that you can move the limb more easily. But massage is not enough—flexibility exercise is also necessary.

Consumer Guide® Rating: Massage is not recommended for the development of physical fitness. Massage is effective for tension release and relief of aching muscles, but its contribution to physical fitness is practically nil. It cannot reduce body fat or weight, and it is not a substitute for active exercise. It is not harmful provided proper techniques are used and you do not have a condition (e.g., varicose veins) that precludes its use. Massage is an acceptable alternative for people who have certain orthopedic conditions and are unable to engage in active exercise.

MASSAGE MACHINES

Massage machines include vibrators, rollers, and whirlpools of various types. Some are comfortable vibrating chairs, others are machines that simulate kneading and stroking movements. Other appliances rely on revolving wooden rollers or vibrating belts to produce light stimulation and relaxation.

Such devices may temporarily relieve muscles that are sore due to unusual exercise or long periods of activity, but don't expect too much. Massage machines provide no easy route to physical fitness.

The late Dr. Arthur Steinhaus, Ph.D., demonstrated that mechanical vibrators are not a legitimate way to remove or redistribute body fat. Steinhaus subjected thirteen men (some markedly overweight) to a fifteen-minute period of vigorous vibration by a belt massager, with the belt around the abdomen. He found they used up about 11.41 extra calories per fifteen-minute bout (about one twenty-third of an ounce of body weight). He also measured blood fat levels and found that there was no increase in the amount of fat circulating in the bloodstream. According to his calculations, one would have to use the vibrator fifteen minutes a day for a full year to lose one pound of fat. (A fifteen-minute walk daily would take off ten pounds in one year!) Steinhaus's conclusion was that "the vibrator is not to be taken seriously as a device to assist in fat reduction or in shifting of fat deposits within the body." [13]

Consumer Guide® Rating: Mechanical massage and vibration devices cannot reduce body fat or weight or increase your fitness level. They can help relieve aching muscles and tension, but they are expensive and not the best means to achieve these goals. Therefore, massage machines cannot be recommended for inclusion in a fitness program.

CELLULITE

Nicole Ronsard is a beauty expert who runs a New York beauty salon. According to her publisher, she is acknowledged as an international authority on cellulite. In her book *Cellulite: Those Lumps, Bumps and Bulges You Couldn't Lose Before,* she told the American public that "orange peel fat"—that ugly, bumpy type—is "cellulite." [14] Cellulite was described as fat that is trapped in the connective tissues, saturated with water and toxic waste.

According to Ronsard, "Cellulite is that fat that you just can't seem to lose. . . . It is a gel-like substance made up of fat, water and waste, trapped in lumpy, immovable pockets just beneath the skin. These pockets of 'fat gone wrong' act like sponges that can absorb amounts of water, blow up and bulge out, resulting in ripples and flabbiness you see." [15]

"Orange peel fat" (a dimpling of the skin) does occur in some individuals:

Visually, fat and cellulite are very different. Regular fat, when squeezed, is smooth in texture. In appearance it does not show any ripples or lumps. . . . If cellulite is present, the skin ripples and looks like orange peel. There is also a characteristic nonsensitivity, not present when you squeeze a noncellulite or simple fat area.

At a more advanced stage, the ripples will become more noticeable without applying any pressure. Tissues will be flabby, and sensitivity no longer present in most cases.[16]

The thesis continues that because cellulite is not simply fat, a low-calorie diet is no solution. On a low-calorie diet fat will decrease, but the cellulite bulges will remain. A diet is needed "that purifies the body of excess water and toxic waste without forcing it to burn fat in unnecessary areas. (The diet usually consists of raw fruits and vegetables, low-fat foods, lean meats, plenty of water, yogurt and dried brewer's yeast. Salt intake is also to be reduced.) This diet avoids those foods that tax an already overburdened system, as they contribute to cellulite formation." [17]

Ronsard and other writers [18] claim that other special techniques must be used to rid the body of cellulite. In addition to a diet, these include exercise; massage; high-pressure water massage (squirting a hose on the fat area); relaxation; deep breathing; and overworking the kidneys, intestines, and sweat glands—which means sauna bathing and consuming lots of natural laxatives and diuretics.

Consumer Guide® regards the cellulite concept as a dubious proposition. This skepticism is shared by many experts in the field. One says, "I could not find a single reference to cellulite in numerous medical physiology texts, or books on adipose tissue. In *Index Medicus,* an index of medical literature, there were only five papers in ten years referring to cellulite, and then they referred to the fat as 'so-called cellulite.' " [19] This writer also reports that "Dr. Philip L. White, director of the AMA's food and nutrition department, calls cellulite a figment of Mme. Ronsard's imagination," and that "Dr. Morton Glenn, past president of the American Nutritional Association, said there was no such thing in medical science." [20]

Doctors David Shepro, Ph.D., and Howard Knuttgen, Ph.D., are not as emphatic but clearly have doubts: "That the cosmetic condition is unique and can be treated specifically is truly open to question, but other than exorbitant fees charged for a cure the authors have no objection to the usual prescription for treatment: plenty of exercise, a balanced diet, massage, sauna, and yoga. We doubt if the prescription will cure cellulite but it certainly will not harm you." [21]

The Ronsard thesis that cellulite is trapped fat in connective tissues may be based on outdated concepts. At one time physiologists thought fat was passive in nature, not involved in the body's energy metabolism. According to Dr. H. E. Wertheimer, M.D., of the Hebrew University Hadassah School and one of the world's greatest authorities on adipose tissue, it was believed that the main function of fat was to insulate the body against heat loss and act as support for other tissue. He explains that this thinking has changed. More recent evidence indicates that fat may be stored in two different types of adipose tissue—one that holds lipids ready for a rather quick turnover into energy and a second in which the fat is eventually turned over into energy but on a much slower basis. In either case the fat does not remain in the cell for an extended period of time.[22]

Orange peel fat appears primarily in inactive people, even people who have dieted for most of their life, but rarely in active people. The key seems to be activity.

Consumer Guide® Rating:

1. Cellulite is just plain fat that has accumulated near the surface of the skin. It is not yet known why the dimpling effect occurs in some people and not in others. Why this fat occurs only in certain body areas even Nicole Ronsard cannot explain. *Consumer Guide®* suggests that it occurs more often in women than in men because American women are encouraged to lead a more sedentary life. This is particularly true during the teen-age and early adult years.

2. The massage that the cellulite people recommend may break tension, but it does not break down fat.

3. The concept of "toxic gas" accumulation in connective tissue is not correct.

4. Several recommendations set forth by the cellulite people are good—exercise, good nutrition, relaxation, and good elimination. Good elimination, for example, is essential

to keep the body's fluids at a proper level. Too much fluid may contribute to the "orange peel" effect.

The cellulite program is not recommended for overall fitness. Even as a weight-control program it falls short. If you want to get rid of fat, including the orange peel kind, you must follow good dietary recommendations and engage in exercise in the target heart rate zone, twenty to thirty minutes four times a week.

FIGURE WRAPPING

Figure wrapping comes in many packages. Some of the most popular are "Shape Wrap," "Body Wrap," "Continental Miracle Wrap," "Swiss Trim," "Insta-trim," "Suddenly Slim," "Suddenly Slenda," and the "Benne Method."

Many outlandish claims are made—"You must lose four to twelve inches first treatment" is just one of many.

In a figure-wrapping treatment, you strip and are measured at predetermined locations on your body, a procedure which may be very difficult to duplicate at home. Usually you do not know the technique for arriving at a certain measurement (whether four inches from shoulder, three above the knee, etc.). Another trick used is holding the tape measure in such a fashion that the customer is not able to read it to verify the measurement recorded by the attendant.

After measuring, you are wrapped mummy fashion from ankle to neck in special tapes that have supposedly been soaked in a "magical solution." Parts of the body that do not need reducing may be omitted from the wrapping. You next put on a rubberized sweat suit with elasticized cuffs and neck to prevent air circulation. You relax in a lounge chair, covered with a blanket, listening to soft music or watching television. At the end of one hour, the tapes and suit are removed and you are remeasured.

Does this work? Dr. Ruth Lindsey concluded that it does not. Dr. Lindsey, professor of health and physical education and recreation at Oklahoma State University, working in cooperation with the American Medical Association and the U.S. Food and Drug Administration, conducted a survey of figure-wrapping salons. The results are disturbing. In the March/April 1972 issue of *Fitness for Living,* Dr. Lindsey stated that the treatment may be risky. She reported the warning of an American Medical Association consultant that the antiperspirant action of the aluminum sulphate in the "magic solution" could produce a heat rash and the magnesium sulphate could produce irritation as well as maceration (softening of the tissues). Dr. Lindsey continues:

> But he [the AMA consultant] believes the greatest risk is the possibility of dehydration and heat exhaustion from the inhibition of heat radiation from the skin while it is sealed in tapes and a sauna suit for an hour. . . . He states: "It would be advisable to have the temperature, pulse, respiration and blood pressure closely monitored by trained medical personnel throughout the period of treatment."[23]

Dr. Lindsey lists a number of chemical solutions that might be used to produce dehydration effects and adds that the pressure of the bandages may also reduce the blood volume of the extremities, diverting it to internal organs and deeper body tissues. Even air conditioning may be a factor: "When the refrigerated air strikes the saturated victim, a chilling effect occurs. Known as hypothermy, the cold produces a constriction of the superficial blood vessels causing an actual temporary reduction in the size of the body parts." [24]

So, Dr. Lindsey concludes, your measurements may actually be reduced by the treatment: "The dehydrating solution, the pressure from the bandages, the vasoconstriction from the cold and perhaps a little cheating with the tape measure can produce 'amazing results'—*temporarily.* None of the effects described would induce permanent changes in the customer's figure." [25]

In a few hours, you'd be back to normal size. Lindsey's conclusions are firm and negative: "There is no chemical substance known to science which can be applied to the body to produce a permanent reducing effect and/or 'react with the fat' to make it disappear. Aside from the possible health hazards described by the AMA consultant, it appears that the efficacy of such a reducing treatment is highly questionable." [26] And again, quite simply: *"There is no way to reduce weight or bulk except through exercise and diet control.* There are no miracles. In the long run, from what we have found, figure wrapping doesn't work." [27]

Consumer Guide® Rating: Figure wrapping is a fraud and should be banned. It does not work and may be dangerous.

19

HEALTH AND FITNESS CENTERS: FANTASY LAND OR ... ?

SOME ARE KNOWN AS HEALTH CLUBS OR SPAS, OTHERS weight-reducing or figure salons, and still others fitness centers.* The facilities range from plush clubs with deep shag carpets and chrome-plated equipment, complete with mirrors and music, to dingy rooms that have seen better days. The programs offered may also be as different as night and day—some very good, some very bad, and a host in between.

COMMERCIAL HEALTH CLUBS

Today health clubs are big business. It is reported that three million Americans pay upward of $300 a year for the privilege of exercising—that's about $900 million a year! [1]

The clubs come in all sizes. Some are small, with only a handful of members at one location, grossing a few thousand

---

* As a very rough rule of thumb, health clubs and fitness centers focus on exercise for fitness with less emphasis on vibrating machines and figure wrapping, etc. Figure salons stress figure wrapping, vibrating machines, and other passive machines, combined with some exercise.

dollars a year. On the other hand, huge chains such as Jack LaLanne, Vic Tanny, Silhouette/American, Holiday Health Spas, Elaine Powers, and European Health Spas have thousands of members and collect mind-boggling annual fees. A quick look at the Yellow Pages under "physical fitness," "gymnasiums," and "weight reducing" will provide a listing of health clubs in your area and give you an idea of how popular health clubs are.

HEALTH CLUB FACILITIES

Most health clubs have a set of chrome-plated weights of various poundages and/or multi-station gyms for muscle strength and muscle endurance. Most have incline boards for abdominal work and other assorted strength machines. Rowing machines, stationary bicycles, and more recently treadmills may be available for development of cardiovascular endurance. (The bicycles and treadmills are a new feature in many clubs and are rapidly gaining popularity.) Roller massagers and vibrating belt massagers that are supposed to roll off fat are extremely popular and are found in practically every club. Automatic massage tables and masseur and masseuse services are also popular. Ultraviolet and infrared lamps are often available in the massage rooms or nearby. Mirrors and padded exercise tables are a must. Many health clubs also offer whirlpool baths and both steam and sauna rooms. Some have small swimming pools. Some of the most up-to-date spas have a small jogging track (twenty-five laps to a mile).

THE HEALTH CLUB PROGRAM

There are probably as many exercise programs as there are clubs. Instructors make their own modifications of the training manuals' plans, which complicates this subject even further. It is safe to say, however, that the major thrust of a health club program is use of the equipment. And the services used most extensively are the muscle strength and endurance equipment, vibrator belts, and rollers. Abdominal work on the slant board is also very popular, and emphasis is often placed on steam and sauna. Up-to-date clubs recommend cardiovascular exercise on the treadmill, bicycle, rowing machine, or jogging track.

In addition to these basics, many clubs offer karate, belly dancing, yoga, swimming, dance exercises, stop-smoking clinics, and weight-control sessions.[2]

People give many different reasons for joining health clubs: the idea of group exercise ("it keeps me motivated"), the convenience ("no need to exercise in outdoor heat or cold"), the plush atmosphere ("I like to pamper myself"), social contacts ("I see my friends there, or I might pick up a date"), the machines ("I'm too lazy to exercise by myself"), the personal attention ("I need to have someone check on my progress"), or the ads ("I've always wanted to try it").

One thing should be clear before we get into detailed evaluation of the health club alternative. A health club is not a necessity for fitness.

CRITICISMS OF COMMERCIAL HEALTH CLUBS AND FIGURE SALONS

Dennis Moore, researcher for the Maryland Center of Public Broadcasting, reviewed health spas and lamented the unsavory tactics adopted by many clubs. He compared the health club promises to the themes used by automobile companies: shiny chrome and sex. "The appeal is so quintessentially American that it may, in fact, be one of the best ways to get a notoriously and dangerously lethargic population out of its chair and into some activity. The problem with some spas is that, along with the chrome and sex, they have adopted the less savory practices of the auto business—the high-pressure sales, one-sided installment contracts, and assorted deceptions which have made the used car dealer the untrustworthy figure he is today." [3]

In an effort to counteract high-pressure tactics, the Federal Trade Commission has proposed regulations to correct the "deceptive and misleading advertising" and sales presentations used by many health spas.[4] The FTC asked some spas to include a three-day trial period in their contract.[5] This gives a consumer time to visit the health spa on a trial basis, reconsider the benefits and costs, and cancel the contract if he or she wishes. If a customer cancels within the stated cooling-off period, all fees must be returned.

The FTC has now made this proposal nationwide, adding a few more stipulations. In addition to the three-day cooling-off period, participants would be able to drop out after beginning a program and still receive at least a partial refund. "The health salons would be able to keep a cancellation fee of up to 5 percent of the total contract price, plus a pro-rated part of the contract price based on the time the facilities were available to the customer for use." [6]

Apparently the FTC agrees with Dennis Moore's charge that there are other "assorted deceptions," for the FTC has issued a list of several unfair practices used by health spas or clubs:

1 / High-pressure sales tactics.
2 / Closing facilities or going out of business without making arrangements to meet their contractual obligations to customers.
3 / Selling membership contracts to customers who are not physically qualified to participate in the activities of the club. (One of the proposed rules would require clubs to inform customers that if they are over thirty-five years of age or have suspected heart disease, they should consult with their doctor before enrolling.)

4 / Offers of fictitious bargains.
5 / Misrepresentation of the facilities available and the qualifications of the employees.
6 / False claims about the effectiveness of weight reduction and figure taping programs.
7 / Unfair cancellation and refund policies.[7]

Another problem is unqualified instructors. Many are merely salespersons. "Too many instructors are hired for their ability to sell you contracts, and their training might have emphasized sales psychology rather than exercise physiology. Instructors should not have to sell." [8]

Another shortcoming of the great majority of clubs is the emphasis on muscle strength and endurance and occasionally an even greater emphasis on rollers, vibrators, and steam treatments. In light of current knowledge and fitness research, this is an inadequate program. As we have stressed in this book, cardio-respiratory fitness is the key to better health.

DR. JIMMY JOHNSON: REBUTTAL

Consumer Guide® asked Dr. Jimmy Johnson, Executive Director of the Association of Physical Fitness Centers (a trade association of full-service health spas), to rebut the criticism lodged against health clubs.

Dr. Johnson describes the sales presentations as "rather elaborate explanations of the pros and cons of the benefits of physical fitness." The object is to create "positive" members, "who know what they're there for, who know the benefits, who understand that the problem of physical fitness lies with them, who comprehend the fact that it is hard work, that they will have to regularly attend the spa and cannot just attend it willy-nilly and achieve results."

Dr. Johnson explains that joining a health club is like

buying a car. You are buying a complete package, and you are paying for it in installments. The monthly charge is *not* a monthly usage figure. The companies would much prefer to receive the total price of the membership in cash when the people sign up, but as a convenience to the customer, as in other industries, the clubs offer sales contracts that allow for payment over two years. "You have to understand that the major costs for the company are incurred while acquiring the member and during the first month after joining. But the return on the investment comes back when these people pay up over a year or two. And remember, there are no long-term contracts in this association any more, unless you consider two years a long time. Lifetime contracts and five-, six-, and eight-year contracts have been abolished."

Johnson acknowledges that you can find people in the spas who do not have a degree in physical education or physical therapy. He explains that many of these people have been trained through in-house training programs—"the same kind of training programs that General Electric gives their people in repairing televisions and the same kind of training that other industries give their employees to deal with specialized activities. Most of these programs are under the supervision of academic experts and professionals."

Johnson also admits, "In the past, emphasis was on muscle strength and muscle endurance. But the trend now is toward cardiovascular fitness. The transition will take time, but the trend is definitely in that direction."

Consumer Guide® Rating: There are exceptions to all generalizations: Some health clubs do an outstanding job and others are frauds or near-frauds. The range can be found among national chains as well as among one-person operations. It is extremely difficult to make blanket statements, but *Consumer Guide*® can at least set down some guidelines.

HIGH-PRESSURE SELLING. When you enter a health club, you can expect a tour followed by a high-pressure sales pitch.

Be ready for it. Instructors and managers are well-schooled in making an effective presentation. They want your business.

Consumer Guide® sees nothing wrong with the health club manager making a strong case emphasizing the value of exercise. But that's it. Under no circumstances should you feel badgered, embarrassed, belittled, threatened, detained, or mocked. If you feel any excessive amount of pressure, leave or at least ask for more time. If you are told this is a once-in-a-lifetime deal or that the rates go up tomorrow, etc., forget it. It's a high-pressure outfit interested in the dollar figure, not yours.

THE CONTRACT. Read the contract carefully. If you want more time, take it. If you feel you should read it at home or want to discuss it with other members of your family or anyone else, do so. If the health club won't permit you to take the contract home, steer clear of that organization. Make sure the contract commits you to no more than two years; one year is preferable. All contracts should provide for a minimum three-day cooling-off period; look for a "use of facility" clause permitting you to use the club during those three days.

KEY CONSIDERATIONS. During the tour, explanation of facilities, and closing, you should be aware of the following:

1. Is there a discussion of your individual problems? This should take place prior to signing the contract. Is there a discussion of your physical limitations, risk factors, and the possibility of stress tests? Do they recommend that you talk to your doctor before you embark on an exercise program?

2. Is the person conducting the tour an instructor, a manager, or what? Does he or she seem to be well trained and not just well built? Ask if he or she is a physical education or physical therapy graduate with additional training in fitness. If not, does the club have an in-service training program emphasizing cardiovascular fitness? Do you

sense that the person has a genuine interest in you? Is he or she able to explain how the machines operate, their value and limitations?

3. Does the spa manager or instructor emphasize cardiovascular fitness, or is the focus on muscle strength and muscle endurance? If the emphasis is on muscle strength and endurance, you can eliminate that club. Be careful—even the official statement of the Association of Physical Fitness Centers notes that "the modern health spa . . . offers programs of physical fitness incorporating concepts of progressive resistance exercise for both sexes. . . ." [9] Progressive resistance exercise is the development of muscle endurance and strength. Remember, the primary focus should be on cardiovascular fitness.

4. Visit the club *at a time of day when you plan to use it.* This is crucial. Every club has a peak-usage time. Waiting in line to run on the treadmill, ride a bicycle, or lift weights can be a serious inconvenience. Consider time and use of facilities as important factors.

5. Before signing anything, talk to several of the people who are exercising (or who have just finished, if you don't want to interrupt their work). If the manager doesn't permit you to do this, cross the club off your list. Ask what they think of the program, what the emphasis is, and whether personal attention is given. Try to find out what the dropout rate is. European Health Spas claims that nearly three fourths of their new members are referrals from other members.[10] If the three-fourths figure is correct—and there is no way to check on it—it would indicate that this chain must be doing something right.

6. Find out how long the club has been in your area. The longer the better, and if under the same management, that's another plus. Approach a new club with caution—especially "pre-opening" sales. There have been cases where con artists have held pre-opening sales for clubs that never opened.

7. Find out if the club belongs to the Association of Physical Fitness Centers. This trade association for full-service health spas is dedicated to upgrading the industry. The Association has established a code of ethics that covers programs, facilities, employees, and consumers' rights.

8. The spa needs you more than you need the spa. Don't forget that. All you need for a solid fitness program is a good pair of shoes and a copy of *Rating the Exercises*. A club is an extra. It can provide you with some social contacts, motivation, and a special place to exercise—if you need these things.

THE NATIONAL YMCA

The granddaddy of all health clubs is the YMCA. Other similar organizations are the YWCA, YMHA, YWHA, and CYO—the Christian Youth Organization. The YMCA national fitness director, Dr. Clayton R. Myers, Ph.D., states that five hundred to six hundred Y's (of a total of around eighteen hundred) have bona fide fitness programs—programs emphasizing cardiovascular fitness. Dr. Myers stated that in 1975, 340,000 different physical education groups were operating, and 124,547 physical fitness tests were administered emphasizing cardiovascular fitness. "Moreover," Myers said, "there is a predicted growth factor of around 20 percent a year on all these figures."

The size of the Y's organization and the number of branches make it impossible to generalize on facilities and personnel. Some have four-million-dollar structures and others storefront space that serves as a base of operations for programs held in other community facilities (churches, schools, fire halls, etc.). Some associations have personnel with Ph.D.'s in exercise physiology, and others employ persons with degrees in fields completely unrelated to physical education, let alone physical fitness.

CRITICISMS

The Y has not been without critics.

1. "The Y is not as plush as a health club," Dr. Jimmy Johnson noted. "Many YMCAs have very limited facilities which sometimes are depressing and dilapidated." Even the National Y recognizes this fact. A senior Y staff member admitted that there are "some Y buildings that I'm ashamed to walk into."

2. Most Y's are located in downtown areas, which keeps many people away from them in the evening.

3. Membership in the YMCA is costly, ranging from seventy dollars to over four hundred dollars. You have to be a Y member to use the facilities. Dr. Johnson believes that health clubs are more reasonable. "I know a company that sells what they call a VIP membership. It costs somewhere between $550 to $650 and covers two years. At the end of two years you're entitled to annual membership renewal at a fee that is guaranteed never to go up. The average renewal fee is around $40 a year. So the cost is quite reasonable since if you took a base figure of $500 and the person belonged for four years the total cost of his membership would be $580— or $145 per year. Now, they can go anytime they want, as many times as they want, twice a day, five days a week, once a week, or once a year. Now if you check the YMCA you will find that you can't get that kind of membership."

4. Occasionally the criticism has been made that a Y has more people than the facilities can hold; the result is overcrowding.

5. The local YMCA does not always live up to the standards set forth on the national level. For example, some Y's have vibrators and rollers available. Some also emphasize muscle strength and muscle endurance rather than cardiovascular endurance. And it is apparent that some Y's

do a poor job of programming. The National Y told *Consumer Guide*®, "Most of our personnel are well trained, but some are not. As a result, there are some Y's that are operating substandard programs."

REBUTTALS

1. It is true that most health clubs have plusher facilities than YMCA's. But plushness does not a program make. When it comes to completeness of exercise facilities, the YMCA wins hands down. Dr. Clayton Myers, National Fitness Director for the YMCA, told *Consumer Guide*® that he believes that the Y's are superior in the facilities that count for fitness:

> The Y usually has a great many more facilities to offer for less money. The average health spa, for example, is just a glorified weight-exercise room, and it's heavily invested in machines requiring such small effort that the exercise value is questionable. Even if the equipment is a good weight resistance model, the focus is on a single aspect of fitness. Many clubs advocate passive exercise devices for sales appeal. At a YMCA, however, the facilities will most often include a running track, a pool large enough to really swim in, gymnasiums, handball and racquetball and squash and basketball courts, plus a weight room.

2. Although it is true that some of the Y buildings are badly in need of repair, this is not the case in most instances. And, of course, appearances do not make a program.

3. The fact that many Y's are located in the downtown area could be considered an advantage rather than a disadvantage. A downtown facility provides a place for the average businessman or -woman to exercise during the working day. It also is accessible by public transportation and is available to serve the inner city population.

YMCAs are scattered in many locations—in cities as well as suburbs. Cleveland, for example, has at least twenty-one branches; Los Angeles, over thirty; and Philadelphia, about twenty.[11]

4. According to Clayton Myers, the average Y cost is much lower than that of a health club in similar locations, and there are no long-term contracts. One year is the rule.

5. The discrepancy between national policy and local practice is a problem shared by all large organizations. Dr. Myers relies on trained personnel to implement programs and has great faith in the Y's internal training program. "Because the National Y has a training program and support system, we have a method for improving professional skills, implementing new programs, and updating ongoing programs. The training that we provide is quite extensive. Workshops, seminars, and conferences are conducted frequently to keep our standards high."

Consumer Guide® Rating: It is our opinion that in most instances a YMCA is preferable to a profit-motivated health club. The hiring practices are better as are the training programs. Other nonprofit organizations—such as the YMHA and YWCA—also probably have better programs and trained personnel. On the other hand, the facilities of these nonprofit organizations are not, in most instances, as plush as those in commercial health clubs. So many criticisms have been lodged against the commercial health clubs, however, that there is reason to expect a greater chance of poorer programs or a "rip-off" than with a nonprofit organization such as the Y.

Consumer Guide® recommends following the guidelines outlined in this chapter before joining any club—profit or nonprofit. Finding the right fitness facility is not a simple task; one must be an astute, well-informed consumer in this market.

20

RATING
THE EXERCISES

EACH RATING IS BASED ON AN EVALUATION OF SELECTED factors *Consumer Guide®* considers vital to a quality fitness program. Those programs which properly emphasize cardiovascular fitness are ranked highest. Other programs are downgraded accordingly. The criteria include primary emphasis on cardiovascular fitness; consideration for flexibility, body composition, muscle strength, and muscle endurance; proper warm-up and cool-down; proper medical clearance and information; logical progression of exercise; variety of exercises; avoidance of potentially harmful exercises; and ease of implementing the program.

FOUR STARS. To be rated four stars a program must recommend activities that are aerobic in nature. It must emphasize the proper intensity (70 percent to 85 percent of maximum heart rate or the equivalent) and duration (fifteen to thirty minutes). Lower-intensity exercise will be adequate if duration is longer. A four-star program must also recommend exercise a minimum of three or four times a week and provide a good and realistic progression of improvement (moving from a low level of fitness to a higher level). Correct information must be given with respect to fitness, exercise physiology, fitness testing, and medical guidance. Although desirable, it is not necessary for the program to include

flexibility, strength, muscle endurance exercises, or a variety
of activities.

Bowerman's and Harris's *Jogging*
Canada's *The Fit Kit*
Cooper's *Aerobics for Women*
Cooper's *The New Aerobics*
Cooper's *The Aerobics Way*
Cureton's *Physical Fitness and Dynamic Health*
deVries' *Vigor Regained*
Fixx's *The Complete Book of Running*
Graham's *Prescription for Life*
Kiell's and Frelinghuysen's *Keep Your Heart Running*
Myers' *Official YMCA Physical Fitness Program*
PCPFS's *Jogging/Running*
PCPFS's *The Fitness Challenge*
Shepro's and Knuttgen's *Complete Conditioning*
Zohman's *Beyond Diet*

THREE STARS. Three-star exercise programs also must
emphasize aerobic activities. For the most part, these programs are rated second best because they are borderline in
one of the following: intensity, duration, or frequency.
Cooper's *Aerobics* program is placed here because *Consumer
Guide*® feels that too much emphasis is placed on the 12-
Minute Run/Walk.

Ald's *Jogging, Aerobics, and Diet*
Åstrand's *Health and Fitness*
Cooper's *Aerobics*
Mitchell's *The Perfect Exercise* (Paul Smith Program)
PCPFS's Men's Program*
PCPFS's Women's Program*
Swengros' *Fitness with Glenn Swengros*

---

* The President's Council on Physical Fitness and Sports program for men and
women deserves to be in this group *only* if the jog/walk sequence is followed. If the
rope skipping or running-in-place exercises are used, these programs qualify for
only two stars.

TWO STARS. Two-star aerobic programs are those which are deficient or excessive in their exercise recommendations. The first three would have scored much higher had they not recommended rather dramatic advances in their progressions. The next two programs did not record enough cardiovascular exercise. These programs also present generally accurate information about cardiovascular fitness.

Johnson's and Bass's *Creative Walking*
Leonard's, Hofer's and Pritkin's *The 2100 Plan*
Mitchell's *The Joy of Jogging*
Mitchell's *The Perfect Exercise* (Rodahl Program)
Rose's and Martin's *The Lazy Man's Guide to Physical Fitness*

The following seven two-star programs focus on muscular fitness with a marginal amount of time spent on cardiovascular fitness (less than ten minutes).

Graham's and Selin's *Physical Fitness for the Business Man*
Lettvin's *The Beautiful Machine*
Miss Craig's 21-Day Shape-up Plan
Prudden's *How to Keep Slender and Fit After 30*
Rodahl's *Be Fit for Life*
Royal Canadian Air Force—XBX
Royal Canadian Air Force—5BX

ONE STAR. One-star aerobic or muscular fitness programs are those that fail to recommend enough exercise. With respect to cardiovascular exercise, they usually come up short in two of the following: intensity, duration, or frequency. In a few instances incorrect information is given about improvement of physical fitness. With respect to muscle fitness, they generally do not provide adequate progressions. For the most part, these are really fruitless programs, except for people who are extremely unfit (such as post-operative). Once an unfit person makes some improvement in these programs, not enough exercise is recommended for continual progress.

> Buster Crabbe's *Energistics*
> Dr. Solomon's *Master Plan for Physical Fitness*
> King's *Golden Age Exercises*
> Metropolitan Life's Exercise Guide—Men
> Metropolitan Life's Exercise Guide—Women
> Morehouse's and Gross's *Total Fitness*
> Spackman's *Exercise in the Office*

The following one-star programs emphasize a single component of fitness other than cardiovascular—either flexibility, muscle strength, or muscle endurance. Although these programs are given only one star, several—*those with an asterisk (*)—are recommended as an adjunct to any four-star program that does not emphasize flexibility or muscle strength.*

> Isokinetic Programs (with isometrics)
> Isokinetic Programs (without isometrics) *
> Isometric Programs
> Weight Training Programs *
> > PCPFS's *Weight Training Program for Strength and Power*
> > Ravelle's *Bodybuilding for Everyone*
> > Reynolds' *Complete Weight Training Book*
> > *Sports Illustrated's Training with Weights*
> > Taylor's *Strength and Stamina Training*
> Yoga Programs *

NO RATING. No rating is given to the two programs that present good information on weight control and exercise but do not provide specific guidelines for exercise other than calorie-burning activities.

> Gwinup's *Energetics*
> Konishi's *Exercise Equivalents of Foods*

NOT RECOMMENDED. *Consumer Guide®* considers the following to be based on completely erroneous concepts of physical fitness and health.

> Cellulite Programs
> Hittleman's *Weight Loss Through Yoga*

RATING OF EXERCISE EQUIPMENT

When considering the purchase of exercise equipment remember that to be effective the product must allow you to be the initiator of the effort. Passive exercise does not work. The following pieces of equipment are rated according to their contribution to cardiovascular fitness. In Chapters 16, 17, and 18 additional information on exercise equipment is provided.

FOUR STARS. Four-star products are those which you can use safely to improve your cardio-respiratory fitness. These products also allow you to make proper adjustments for adequate intensity, duration, and frequency of exercise.

> Jump ropes
> Motorized treadmills
> Nonmotorized bicycles

THREE STARS. Three-star products are those which you can use safely to improve your cardiovascular fitness. These devices, however, have limited applications.

> Creeping devices
> Nonmotorized treadmills
> Rowing machines

ONE STAR. One-star products are those which can be used to improve selected components of physical fitness. The components improved are muscle strength and muscle endurance. To achieve a one-star rating the device must allow you to measure rates of improvement easily and to make adjustments for same.

> Isokinetic products
> Mini-gyms
> Weight training equipment

NOT RECOMMENDED. Products which are not recommended are those which are potentially hazardous or of little value in improving fitness.

> Body trimmers
> Chest pulls
> Exercise wheels
> Motorized bicycles
> Rollers
> Rope stretchers
> Rubberized sweat suits
> Sauna shorts
> Sauna and steamrooms
> Vibrators
> Whirlpools

RATING THE SPORTS

Each sport rating is based on its contribution to the most important component of physical fitness—cardiovascular fitness. It is also assumed that the sport is played a minimum of three times a week (nonconsecutive days) and the players are of equal ability, skill, and fitness level. Please read Chapter 15—How Your Favorite Sport Rates As Exercise—for more information.

FOUR STARS. To be rated four stars a sport must be aerobic in nature. While exercising, your heart rate must be in the *70 percent to 85 percent of maximum* range and you must play *continuously* for at least fifteen to thirty minutes. A four-star program is unique, however, since it also permits you to measure the distance covered. In other words, you can measure progress week after week and month after month.

> Bicycling (11 mph)
> Jogging/Running
> Swimming
> Walking (4½ mph)
> Cross-country Skiing

THREE STARS. To be rated three stars a sport must be aerobic in nature. It is assumed that while participating your heart rate is in the 70 percent to 85 percent of maximum range and that you play *continuously* for at least fifteen to thirty minutes. These activities are ranked second best simply because they make it difficult to measure progress.

> Badminton (singles)
> Basketball
> Bicycling (8 mph)
> Handball
> Ice/Roller Skating *
> Racquetball
> Skiing (downhill)—15-minute runs
> Squash
> Tennis (singles)
> Volleyball

TWO STARS. To be rated two stars a sport must be aerobic in nature. It is assumed that while participating your heart rate is in the 50 percent to 70 percent of maximum heart rate range and that you play continually for at least fifteen minutes.

> Badminton (doubles or recreational)
> Tennis (doubles, or recreational)
> Walking (3½ mph)
> Water Skiing

---

* If distance is measured, these can be ranked as four-star.

ONE STAR. To be rated one star a sport must be aerobic in nature. During participation the heart rate is elevated, but most of the time it is below 50 percent of maximum range. The activity, however, is sustained—thirty minutes or more.

Bicycling (5 mph)
Golf (no cart)
Walking (3 mph)

These are activities that do not provide any cardiovascular benefit.

Bowling
Golf (in a cart)
Softball

NOTES AND SOURCES

Chapter 1

1. *The Sporting Goods Manager.* 1976, Chicago: National Sporting Goods Association, 1976.
2. C. C. Conrad, *Physical Conditioning Through Water Exercises,* Washington, DC: President's Council on Physical Fitness and Sports, no date, p. 1.
3. "How America Gets in Shape," *Datsun Action,* Issue No. 1, 1976, p. 10.
4. C. R. Myers, "The Nationwide YMCA Cardiovascular Health Program," *The Journal of Physical Education,* Summer, 1976, p. 141.
5. "National Adult Physical Fitness Survey," *The President's Council on Physical Fitness and Sports Newsletter,* May, 1973.
6. *Ibid.*
7. *Ibid.*
8. L. E. Morehouse and L. Gross, *Total Fitness.* NY: Simon & Schuster, 1975, p. 18.
9. P.-O. Åstrand, *Health and Fitness.* Ottawa: Information Canada, 1975, p. 8.
10. "Dr. Kenneth H. Cooper: Views from the Aerobics Center," in B. Anderson, (ed.), *SportSource.* Mountain View, CA: World Publications, 1975, p. 22.

11. "Exploring the Frontiers of Fitness Knowledge," *The Physician and Sportsmedicine,* May, 1976, p. 108.

12. J. Ahrends, "American Lifestyle," *The Michigan Journal for Health, Physical Education, and Recreation,* October, 1976, p. 12.

13. H. Kraus and W. Raab, *Hypokinetic Disease.* Springfield, IL: Charles C. Thomas, 1961.

14. J. L. Steinfeld, "Health Conscious Citizens Are a National Asset," *Journal of Physical Education,* March/April, 1972, p. 102.

15. *Heart Facts.* New York: American Heart Association, 1974, pp. 17–18.

16. S. M. Fox and W. L. Haskell, "Population Studies," *Canadian Medical Association Journal,* 96:1967, pp. 806–810.

17. J. Mayer, *Overweight: Causes, Cost and Control.* Englewood Cliffs, NJ: Prentice-Hall, 1968, p. 82.

18. H. Kraus, "Diagnosis and Treatment of Low Back Pain," *General Practitioner,* 5:1952, pp. 88–92.

19. *Hypokinetic Disease, op. cit.,* p. 19.

20. P. D. White, "Health," in C. T. Kuntzleman (ed.), *The Physical Fitness Encyclopedia.* Emmaus, PA: Rodale Press, 1970, pp. 214–215.

21. H. A. deVries and G. M. Adams, "Electromyographic Comparison of Single Doses of Exercise and Meprobamate As to the Effects on Muscular Relaxation," *American Journal of Physical Medicine,* 51:1972, pp. 130–141.

22. R. H. Driscoll, "Exertion Therapy: Rapid Anxiety Reduction Using Physical Exertion and Positive Imagery." Boulder: University of Colorado (Ph.D. dissertation), 1973.

23. *Physical Fitness in Business and Industry.* Washington, DC: The President's Council on Physical Fitness and Sports, no date, p. 5.

24. "The Science of Fitness," *Fitness For Living,* September/October, 1969, p. 77.

25. A. H. Ismail and L. E. Trachtman, "Jogging the Imagination," *Psychology Today,* April, 1973, pp. 78–88.

26. F. W. Kasch, "The Effects of Exercise on the Aging Process," *The Physician and Sportsmedicine,* June, 1976, p. 68.

27. F. Baekeland, "Exercise Deprivation," *Archives of General Psychiatry,* April, 1970, pp. 368–369.

Chapter 2

1. The President's Council on Physical Fitness and Sports, *Physical Fitness Digest,* 1:1971, p. 1.
2. G. A. Sheehan, *Dr. Sheehan on Running.* Mountain View, CA: World Publications, 1975, p. 127.
3. C. T. Kuntzleman, "Can You Pass This Fitness Test?" *Fitness For Living,* January/February, 1972, p. 33.
4. C. T. Kuntzleman, *Activetics.* NY: Peter H. Wyden, 1975, p. 47.
5. F. Heinzleman and R. W. Bagley, "Response to Physical Activity Programs and Their Effect on Health Behavior," *Public Health Reports,* 85:1970, p. 905.

Chapter 3

1. K. H. Cooper, "Guidelines in the Management of the Exercising Patient," *Journal of the American Medical Association,* March 9, 1970, pp. 1663–1664.
2. Sheehan, *op. cit.,* pp. 126–127.
3. "Dr. Kenneth H. Cooper: Views from the Aerobics Center," *op. cit.,* p. 29.
4. F. W. Kasch, Ph.D., San Diego State University, Exercise Physiology Laboratory, personal communication, 1974.
5. *Ibid.*
6. K. H. Cooper, *The New Aerobics.* NY: Bantam Books, 1972, pp. 31–32.
7. A. Keys and J. Brozek, "Body Fat in Adult Men," *Physiological Reviews,* 33:1953, p. 245.
8. *Skinfolds, Body Girths, Biachromial Diameter, and Selected Anthropometric Indices of Adults.* Washington, DC: U.S. Government Printing Office (PHS Publication Pub. No. 1000), Series 11, Number 35, 1970, p. 2.

9. P. E. Allsen, J. M. Harrison, and B. Vance, *Fitness for Life.* Dubuque, IA: Wm. C. Brown, 1976, p. 66.
10. C. R. Myers, *The Official YMCA Physical Fitness Handbook.* NY: Popular Library, 1975, pp. 103–104.
11. *Ibid.*
12. C. R. Myers, L. A. Golding, and W. E. Sinning, eds., *The Y's Way To Physical Fitness.* Emmaus, PA: Rodale Press, 1973, p. 48.
13. H. Kraus and R. P. Hirschland, "Minimum Muscular Fitness Tests in School Children," *Research Quarterly,* May, 1954, p. 178.
14. *Ibid.*
15. Modified and adapted from: *The Official YMCA Physical Fitness Handbook, op. cit.,* p. 106.

Chapter 4

---

1. M. L. Pollock, "Quantification of Endurance Training Programs," in *Exercise and Sports Sciences Reviews,* J. Wilmore, ed., Vol. I. NY: Academic Press, 1973, p. 155. Also, American College of Sports Medicine, *Guidelines for Graded Exercise Testing and Exercise Prescription.* Philadelphia, PA: Lea & Febiger, 1975, pp. 28, 46.
2. L. R. Zohman, *Beyond Diet: Exercise Your Way To Fitness and Heart Health.* Englewood Cliffs, NJ: CPC International, Inc., 1974, p. 19.
3. American Heart Association Committee on Exercise, *Exercise Testing and Training of Apparently Healthy Individuals: A Handbook for Physicians.* NY: American Heart Association, 1972, p. 4.
4. *Activetics, op. cit.,* pp. 134–136.
5. Zohman, *op. cit.,* p. 11.
6. *Ibid.*
7. *Ibid.,* pp. 11–15.
8. *Total Fitness, op. cit.*
9. T. Bassler, "Marathon Running and Immunity to Heart Disease," *The Physician and Sportsmedicine,* April, 1975, p. 77.

10. L. E. Morehouse, "Responses of Men to Heart Exercise Regimens," PO-2-1967, U.S. Public Health Service, Washington, DC, 1966.

11. Bassler, *op. cit.,* p. 44.

12. American College of Sports Medicine, *op. cit.,* p. 43.

13. J. H. Wilmore and R. J. Barnard, "Total Fitness in 30 Minutes a Week" (book review), *Medicine and Science in Sports,* 8:1976, p. ix.

14. Bassler, *op. cit.,* p. 77.

15. "You Can Run Down Running, But ... Bikers Are Hit by Cars and Swimmers Drown," *The Physician and Sportsmedicine,* April, 1975, p. 86.

16. *Activetics, op. cit.,* p. 78.

17. H. Roskamm, "Optimum Patterns of Exercise for Healthy Adults," *Canadian Medical Association Journal,* 96:1967, p. 895.

18. R. J. Shephard, "Intensity, Duration, and Frequency of Exercise Determinance of the Response to a Training Regimen," *Internationale Zeitschrift für Angewandte Physiologie,* 26:1968, p. 272.

19. Zohman, *op. cit.,* p. 19.

20. American Heart Association Committee on Exercise, *op. cit.,* p. 5.

21. M. L. Pollock, T. K. Cureton, and L. Greninger, "Effects of Frequency of Training on Working Capacity, Cardiovascular Function, and Body Composition of Adult Men," *Medicine and Science in Sports,* 1:1969, p. 70.

22. C. T. Kuntzleman, "Effect of Intensity, Total Work, and Frequency on Selected Cardiovascular and Skin-fold Measurements in Middle-Aged Men," Philadelphia, PA: Temple University (unpublished Ed. D. dissertation), 1976.

23. *Fitness For Life, op. cit.,* p. 66.

24. G. Sheehan, "Make '76 the Year of the Magic Six," *The Physician and Sportsmedicine,* January, 1976, p. 29.

25. C. T. Kuntzleman, *Fitness With Fun.* Spring Arbor, MI: Fitness Finders, for the National Council of YMCAs, 1976, p. 7.

26. Morehouse and Gross, *op. cit.,* pp. 192–193.

Chapter 5

1. M. McGee, "Don't Quit," *Fitness For Living,* January/February, 1973, p. 32.
2. A. S. Lewis, "Body Type," in *The Physical Fitness Encyclopedia, op. cit.,* pp. 57–59.
3. W. H. Sheldon, S. Stevens, and W. D. Tucker, *The Varieties of Human Physique.* NY: Harper and Row, 1940.
4. T. K. Cureton, *Physical Fitness Appraisal and Guidance.* St. Louis: C. V. Mosby Co., 1947, p. 70.
5. *Ibid.,* p. 112.
6. P. D. White and C. Mitchell, *Fitness for the Whole Family.* Garden City, NY: Doubleday, 1964, p. 20.
7. H. deVries, *Vigor Regained.* Englewood Cliffs, NJ: Prentice-Hall, 1974.
8. J. P. Wilmore, "Exploding the Myth of Female Inferiority," *The Physician and Sportsmedicine,* May, 1974, p. 54; and S. L. Higgs, "For Better Female Athletes, It's All in the Training," *The Physician and Sportsmedicine,* July, 1974, p. 47.
9. Wilmore, *op. cit.,* p. 58.
10. *Ibid.*

Chapter 6

1. *Heart Facts, op. cit.,* p. 17.
2. J. N. Morris and P. A. B. Raffle, "Coronary Heart Disease in Transport Workers," *British Journal of Industrial Medicine,* 11:1954, p. 260.
3. O. F. Hedley, "Analysis of 5,116 Deaths Reported As Due to Coronary Occlusion in Philadelphia," *U.S. Weekly Public Health Reports,* 54:1959, p. 972.
4. H. L. Taylor, "Coronary Heart Disease in Physically Active and Sedentary Populations," *Journal of Sports Medicine and Physical Fitness,* 2:1962, p. 73.
5. W. B. Kannel, P. Sorlie, and P. McNamara, "The Relation of Physical Activity to Risk of Coronary Heart Disease: The

Framingham Study," in O. A. Larsen and R. O. Malborg (eds.), *Coronary Heart Disease and Physical Fitness.* Baltimore: University Park Press, 1971, p. 256.

6. R. S. Paffenbarger, M. E. Laughlin, A. S. Gima, and R. A. Black, "Work Activity of Longshoremen As Related to Death from Coronary Heart Disease and Stroke," *New England Journal of Medicine,* 20:1970, p. 1109.

7. D. M. Spain, "Occupational Physical Exertion and Coronary Atherosclerotic Heart Disease," *Journal of Occupational Medicine,* February, 1961, p. 54.

8. R. S. Paffenbarger and W. E. Hale, "Work Activity and Coronary Heart Mortality," *New England Journal of Medicine,* 292:1975, p. 545.

9. J. N. Morris, C. Adams, S. P. W. Chave, C. Sirey, and D. J. Sheehan, "Vigorous Exercise in Leisure-Time and the Incidence of Coronary Heart Disease," *The Lancet,* 285:1973, p. 333.

10. *Ibid.*

11. S. M. Fox, "Relationship of Activity Habits to Coronary Heart Disease," in J. P. Naughton and H. K. Hellerstein (eds.), *Exercise Testing and Exercise Training in Coronary Heart Disease.* NY: Academic Press, 1974, pp. 12–13.

12. *Ibid.*

13. *Ibid.*

14. *Ibid.,* pp. 13–14.

15. T. K. Cureton, *Physiological Effects of Exercise Programs on Adults.* Springfield, IL: Charles C. Thomas, 1969, p. 52.

16. D. Gsell and J. Mayer, "Low Blood Cholesterol Associated with High Calorie, High Saturated-Fat Intakes in a Swiss Alpine Village Population," *American Journal of Clinical Nutrition,* 10:1962, p. 471.

17. J. L. Boyer and F. W. Kasch, "Exercise Therapy in Hypertensive Men," *Journal of American Medical Association,* 211:1668–1671, March 9, 1970.

18. K. H. Cooper, M. L. Pollock, R. P. Martin, S. R. White, A. C. Linnerud, and A. Jackson, "Physical Fitness Levels Versus Selected Coronary Risk Factors," *Journal of American Medical Association,* July 12, 1976, p. 166.

Chapter 7

1. National Research Council, *Recommended Dietary Allowances.* Revised 1948, Reprint and Circular Series, No. 129, Washington, DC, 1948.
2. J. Mayer, N. B. Marshall, J. J. Vitale, J. H. Christensen, M. B. Mashayekhi, and F. J. Stare, "Exercise, Food Intake and Body Weight in Normal Rats and Genetically Obese Adult Mice," *American Journal of Physiology,* 177:1954, p. 544.
3. J. Mayer, P. Roy, and K. P. Mitia, "Relation Between Caloric Intake, Body Weight and Physical Work: Studies in Industrial Male Population in West Bengal," *American Journal of Clinical Nutrition,* 4:1956, p. 169.
4. *Overweight: Causes, Cost, and Control, op. cit.,* p. 20; and J. Mayer, "The Ventromedial Glucostatic Mechanism As a Component of Satiety," *Postgraduate Medicine,* 38:1965, p. 101.
5. J. Mayer, "Obesity: Etiology and Pathogenesis," *Postgraduate Medicine,* 25:1959, p. 267.
6. H. Bruch, *Eating Disorders.* NY: Basic Books, Inc., 1973, pp. 54–58.
7. A. J. Stunkard, "The Management of Obesity," *New York State Journal of Medicine,* 58:1958, p. 79.
8. B. Zuti and L. Golding, "Comparing Diet and Exercise As Weight Reduction Tools," *The Physician and Sportsmedicine,* January, 1976, p. 49.

Chapter 8

1. K. H. Cooper, *Aerobics.* NY: M. Evans, 1968.
2. T. K. Cureton, *Physical Fitness and Dynamic Health.* NY: Dial Press, 1965.
3. Time-Life Editors, *The Healthy Life.* NY: Time-Life, 1966.
4. M. Graham, *Prescription for Life.* NY: David H. McKay, 1966.

5. W. J. Bowerman and W. E. Harris, *Jogging.* NY: Grosset and Dunlap, 1967.

6. *Aerobics, op. cit.*

7. K. H. Cooper, *The New Aerobics.* NY: Bantam Books, 1970.

8. M. Cooper and K. H. Cooper, *Aerobics for Women.* NY: Bantam Books, 1972.

9. K. H. Cooper, *Aerobics.* NY: Bantam Books, 1968.

10. *Ibid.,* p. 22.

11. *The New Aerobics op. cit.,* pp. 22–23, 27.

12. *Ibid.,* pp. 25–26.

13. *Aerobics for Women, op. cit.,* p. 61.

14. "Dr. Kenneth Cooper: Views from the Aerobics Center," *op. cit.,* p. 22.

15. "Run For Your Life?" *The Wall Street Journal,* Wednesday, September 3, 1975, p. 1.

16. *Ibid.*

17. M. Friedman and R. H. Rosenman, *Type A Behavior and Your Heart.* NY: Fawcett World Library, 1973, p. 149.

18. "Run For Your Life?" *op. cit.,* p. 1.

19. *Dr. Sheehan on Running, op. cit.,* pp. 26–27.

20. J. Massie, A. Rode, T. Skrien, and R. J. Shephard, "A Critical Review of the 'Aerobics' Point System," *Medicine and Science in Sports,* Spring, 1970, p. 6.

21. *Ibid.,* p. 6.

22. F. Vitale, *Individualized Fitness Programs.* Englewood Cliffs, NJ: Prentice-Hall, 1973, pp. 130–132.

23. L. E. Morehouse and L. Gross, *Total Fitness.* NY: Pocket Books, 1975, pp. 136–137.

24. T. K. Cureton, "The Comparison of Various Types of Improvements Brought About by Diverse Programs (Tensive, Games, Short-Duration Type vs. Longer, Rhythmic Type) in Physical Fitness Work With Adults," American College of Sports Medicine Meeting, Atlanta, GA, May, 1969.

25. T. K. Cureton, "The Role of Exercise in Health and Fitness," *American Corrective Therapy Journal,* March/April, 1976, p. 12.

26. S. A. Plowman and T. K. Cureton, "Training Effects in Young Adult Women, A Comparison of Continuous, Rhythmical Group Programs and an Individualized 'Aerobic' Type Points

Program," *American Corrective Therapy Journal,* September/October, 1973, pp. 45–50.

27. "Physical Fitness Levels vs. Selected Coronary Risk Factors," *op. cit.,* July 12, 1976, pp. 166–169.
28. Vitale, *loc. cit.*
29. Cooper *et al., loc. cit.*
30. *Aerobics for Women, op. cit.,* pp. 35–36.
31. "Prescription: Run or Jog," *The Physician and Sportsmedicine,* April, 1976, p. 98.
32. H. Johnson and R. Bass, *Creative Walking For Physical Fitness.* NY: Grosset and Dunlap, 1970.
33. *Ibid.,* pp. 32–34.
34. *Ibid.,* p. 34.
35. M. L. Pollock, H. S. Miller, R. Janeway, A. C. Linnerud, B. Robertson, and R. Valentino, "Effects of Walking on Body Composition and Cardiovascular Function of Middle-Aged Men," *Journal of Applied Physiology,* January, 1971, pp. 126–130.
36. *Ibid.,* p. 127.
37. *Jogging,* p. 4.
38. G. A. Sheehan, "Diseases of Excellence," *Fitness For Living,* November/December, 1973, pp. 26–31.
39. W. G. Clancy, "Lower Extremity Injuries in the Jogger and Distance Runner," *The Physician and Sportsmedicine,* June, 1974, pp. 47–50.
40. "Foot Problems in Runners," *The Physician and Sportsmedicine,* July, 1976, pp. 29–45.
41. J. I. Seder, "Heel Injuries Incurred in Running and Jogging," *The Physician and Sportsmedicine,* October, 1976, pp. 70–73.
42. S. D. Fordham, "Stress Fractures Affect Variety of Exercises," *The Physician and Sportsmedicine,* November, 1976, pp. 79–82.
43. *First Steps to Fitness.* Mountain View, CA: World Publications, 1974, p. 36.
44. *Ibid.;* and "Foot Problems in Runners," *op. cit.*
45. G. A. Sheehan, "In Preventative Conditioning, Consider Yoga," *The Physician and Sportsmedicine,* November, 1973, p. 17.
46. *Type A Behavior and Your Heart, op. cit.,* pp. 148 and 156.
47. "You Can Run Down Running, But ... Bikers Are Hit By

Cars and Swimmers Drown," *The Physician and Sports-medicine,* April, 1975, p. 6.

48. E. G. Schmidt, "Jogging Can Kill You," *Playboy,* March, 1976, pp. 87, 152, 153.
49. "You Can Run Down Running, But ... Bikers Are Hit by Cars and Swimmers Drown," *op. cit.,* p. 93.
50. *Ibid.,* pp. 87–89.
51. *Ibid.,* p. 86.
52. J. S. Skinner, "View Point: The Mis-Information Crisis," *American College of Sports Medicine Bulletin,* January, 1977, p. 6.
53. *Type A Behavior and Your Heart, op. cit.,* p. 183.
54. G. A. Sheehan, "Exercise for Fun," *Family Weekly,* January 22, 1977, p. 6.
55. "Prescription: Run or Jog," pp. 93–98; and "Exertion Therapy: Rapid Anxiety Reduction Using Physical Therapy and Positive Imagery," *op. cit.*
56. "You Can Run Down Running, But ... Bikers Are Hit by Cars and Swimmers Drown," *op. cit.,* p. 92.
57. *Ibid.,* p. 86.
58. C. Mitchell, *The Joy of Jogging.* NY: Rutledge Books and Ace News Company, 1968.
59. *Ibid.,* p. 79.
60. *President's Council on Physical Fitness and Sports Jogging/Running Guidelines.* Washington, DC: U. S. Government Printing Office. No date.
61. *Ibid.,* p. 5.
62. *Ibid.*
63. J. L. Leonard, J. L. Hofer, and N. Pritikin, *Live Longer Now.* NY: Grosset and Dunlap, 1974.
64. *Ibid.,* p. 181.

Chapter 9

1. *Total Fitness,* Pocket Books, *op. cit.,* p. 30.
2. *Ibid.,* p. 177.
3. *Ibid.,* p. 178.
4. *Ibid.,* p. 177.

5. *Ibid.*
6. *Ibid.*
7. "Exploring the Frontiers of Fitness Knowledge," *op. cit.,* p. 108.
8. *Ibid.*
9. "Total Fitness in 30 Minutes a Week," (book review), *op. cit.,* p. ix.
10. "No Sweat Exercise Is a Sweaty Issue," *National Observer,* July 1, 1975, p. 1.
11. *Ibid.*
12. *Ibid.*
13. *Total Fitness,* Pocket Books, *op. cit.,* p. 30.
14. "Exploring the Frontiers of Fitness Knowledge," *op. cit.*
15. L. E. Morehouse, "Letter to the Editor," *American College of Sports Medicine Bulletin,* October, 1976, p. 10.
16. M. Flint, B. Drinkwater, and S. Horvath, "Effects of Training on Women's Response to Submaximal Exercise," *Medicine and Science in Sports,* 6: 89–94, 1974; E. A. Harris and B. B. Porter, "On the Heart Rate During Exercise, The Esophageal Temperature and Oxygen Debt," *Quarterly Journal of Experimental Physiology,* 43: 313–319, 1958; and "Response of Men to a Heart Exercise Regimen," *loc. cit.*
17. L. E. Morehouse, "Letter to the Editor," *loc. cit.*
18. B. L. Drinkwater, "Letter to the Editor," *American College of Sports Medicine Bulletin,* January, 1977, p. 2.
19. J. Wilmore and R. J. Barnard, "Letter to the Editor," *American College of Sports Medicine Bulletin,* October, 1976, p. 10.
20. "No Sweat Exercise Is a Sweaty Issue," *op. cit.,* p. 1.
21. *Beyond Diet: Exercise Your Way to Fitness and Heart Health,* *op. cit.,* p. 9.
22. *Prescription for Life, op. cit.,* pp. 89–90.
23. *Ibid.,* p. 91.
24. R. Ald, *Jogging, Aerobics and Diet.* NY: New American Library, 1968.
25. C. Mitchell, *The Perfect Exercise.* NY: Simon & Schuster, 1976.
26. *Ibid.,* p. 72.

Chapter 10

1. *The Official YMCA Physical Fitness Handbook, loc. cit.*
2. N. Solomon and E. Harrison, *Dr. Solomon's Proven Master Plan for Total Body Fitness and Maintenance.* NY: Putnam, 1976, p. 30.
3. *Physical Fitness and Dynamic Health, loc. cit.*
4. W. T. White, "Exercise To Keep Fit," *Sports Illustrated,* January 18, 1955, p. 63.
5. *Physical Fitness and Dynamic Health, op. cit.,* pp. 75–76.
6. *Ibid.,* p. 90.
7. *The Official YMCA Physical Fitness Handbook,* p. 75.
8. *Physical Fitness and Dynamic Health,* p. 90.
9. P.-O. Åstrand, *Health and Fitness.* Stockholm: Skandia Insurance Company, 1973.
10. *Health and Fitness, loc. cit.*
11. *Ibid.,* p. 6.
12. *Ibid.,* p. 54.
13. D. Shepro and H. G. Knuttgen, *Complete Conditioning: The No-Nonsense Guide to Fitness and Good Health.* Reading, MA: Addison-Wesley, 1975.
14. P. J. Kiell and J. S. Frelinghuysen, *Keep Your Heart Running.* NY: Winchester Press, 1976.
15. *Ibid.,* p. 120.
16. *Ibid.,* p. 122.
17. *The Fit Kit.* Ottawa: Recreation Canada, 1975.
18. K. Rodahl, *Be Fit for Life.* NY: Harper & Row, 1966.
19. K. D. Rose and J. D. Martin, *The Lazy Man's Guide to Physical Fitness.* Chicago, IL: Greatlakes Living Press, 1974, p. 28.
20. "Exploring the Effects of Exercise on Hypertension," *The Physician and Sportsmedicine,* December, 1976, p. 46.
21. B. Crabbe, *Energistics.* Chicago, IL: Playboy Press, 1976.

Chapter 11

1. P. J. Rasch and F. L. Allman, "Controversial Exercises," *American Corrective Therapy Journal*, July/August, 1972, p. 95.
2. A. J. Ryan, "Hazardous Exercises" (letter to the editor), *Fitness For Living*, September/October, 1970, p. 5.
3. C. T. Kuntzleman, "Dangerous Exercise, Which, When and Why," *Fitness For Living*, January/February, 1971, p. 25.
4. "Controversial Exercises," *op. cit.*, p. 96.
5. *Ibid.*
6. *Ibid.*
7. "Dangerous Exercise, Which, When and Why," p. 26.
8. K. Klein, "The Deep Squat Exercise as Utilized in Weight Training for Athletics and Its Effects on the Ligaments of the Knee," *Journal of the Association of Physical and Mental Rehabilitation*, 15:1961, p. 6.
9. "Controversial Exercises," *op. cit.*, p. 96.
10. "Hazardous Exercises," *op. cit.*, p. 5.
11. *Ibid.*, p. 6.
12. *Activetics, op. cit.*, pp. 134–135.
13. *Ibid.*, p. 124.
14. "Exercises," in *The Physical Fitness Encyclopedia, op. cit.*, p. 155.
15. *Royal Canadian Air Force, Exercise Plans for Physical Fitness.* NY: Pocket Books, 1975.
16. *Individualized Fitness Programs, op. cit.*, p. 134.
17. *Ibid.*
18. President's Council on Physical Fitness, *Adult Physical Fitness.* Washington, DC: U.S. Government Printing Office, 1965.
19. *Metropolitan Life's Exercise Guide.* NY: Metropolitan Life Insurance Company, 1966.
20. B. Prudden, *How to Keep Slender and Fit After Thirty.* NY: Pocket Books, Inc., 1970, p. 71.
21. *Ibid.*, p. 272.
22. M. Craig, *Miss Craig's 21-Day Shape-Up Program for Men and Women.* NY: Random House, 1968.

23. N. Solomon and M. Knudson, *Dr. Solomon's Easy, No-Risk Diet.* NY: Coward, McCann & Geoghegan, 1974.
24. N. Solomon and E. Harrison, *Doctor Solomon's Proven Master Plan for Total Body Fitness and Maintenance.* NY: Putnam, 1976, pp. 21–22.
25. M. Lettvin, *The Beautiful Machine.* NY: Alfred A. Knopf, 1973.
26. G. Swengros and J. J. Monteleone, *Fitness With Glenn Swengros.* NY: Hawthorne Books, Inc., 1971.

Selected Yoga Books

1. R. Bender, *Stay Young and Flexible After 50.* Ruben Publishing, 1976.
2. R. Bender, *Yoga Exercises for Every Body.*
3. R. Carr, *The Yoga Way to Release Tension.* NY: Barnes and Noble, 1975.
4. W. A. Compton, *Hathayoga.* NY: Harper and Row, 1975.
5. H. Day, *Executive Yoga.* NY: Pinnacle Books.
6. I. Devi, *Yoga for Americans.* Englewood Cliffs, NJ: Prentice-Hall, Inc., 1959.
7. I. Devi, *Forever Young, Forever Healthy.* Englewood Cliffs, NJ: Prentice-Hall, Inc., 1953.
8. R. Hittleman, *Introduction to Yoga.* NY: Bantam Books, 1969.
9. R. Hittleman, *Be Young with Yoga.* NY: Warner Books, 1962.
10. R. Hittleman, *Richard Hittleman's Yoga 28-Day Exercise Plan.* Workman Publishing Co., 1969.
11. R. Hittleman, *Weight Control Through Yoga.* NY: Bantam Books, 1971.
12. R. Hittleman, *Guide to Yoga Meditation.* NY: Bantam Books, 1964.
13. I. Jackson, *Yoga and the Athlete.* Mountain View, CA: World Publications, 1975.
14. N. Phelan and M. Volin, *Yoga for Women.* NY: Harper and Row, 1964.
15. E. Rawls and E. Diskin, *Yoga for Beauty and Health: Look Younger and Be Relaxed.* NY: Warner Books, 1974.

16. S. Richmond, *How to Be Healthy with Yoga.* NY: Arc Books, 1966.
17. R. B. Simon, *Relax and Stretch.* NY: Macmillan, 1975.
18. J. Stern, *Yoga, Youth and Reincarnation.* NY: Bantam Books, 1970.
19. S. Vishnudevananda, *The Complete Illustrated Book of Yoga.* NY: Bell Pub. Co., 1970.
20. M. Volin and N. Phelan, *Yoga for Beauty.* NY: Arc Books, 1966.
21. A. T. Webb, *Slimming with Yoga.* NY: Pocket Books, 1970.
22. E. Wood, *Yoga.* Middlesex, England: Penguin Books, 1972.
23. S. Yesudian and E. Haich, *Yoga and Health.* NY: Harper and Row, 1965.
24. F. R. Young, *Yoga for Men Only.* Englewood Cliffs, NJ: Prentice-Hall, 1969.

Chapter 12

1. A. Ryan, "Yoga and Fitness," *Journal of Health, Physical Education, and Recreation,* February, 1971, p. 26.
2. I. Devi, *Yoga for Americans.* NY: The New American Library, 1961, p. xxxii.
3. J. Haberern, "Yoga," in *The Physical Fitness Encyclopedia, op. cit.,* p. 560.
4. R. Hittleman, *Be Young with Yoga.* NY: Warner Books, Inc., 1975, pp. 5–6.
5. R. Hittleman, "Give Your Back a Break—Try Yoga," *Family Health,* September, 1974, pp. 46–47.
6. H. A. deVries, *The Physiology of Exercise for Physical Education and Athletics.* Dubuque, IA: William C. Brown, 1966, pp. 258–267 and 360–370.
7. "In Preventative Conditioning, Consider Yoga," *op. cit.,* p. 17.
8. "Yoga and Fitness," *op. cit.,* p. 27.
9. W. F. Updyke and P. B. Johnson, *Principles of Modern Physical Education, Health, and Recreation.* NY: Holt, Rinehart, and Winston, 1970, pp. 569–570.
10. N. G. Alexiou, "Yoga—Style, Relaxation, and Advice for the Elderly," *Family Practice News,* March 1, 1973, p. 24.

11. B. W. Anand, G. S. Chhina, and B. Singh, "Some Aspects of Electroencephalographic Studies in Yogis," *Electroencephalography and Clinical Neurophysiology,* 13, 1961, pp. 452–456; B. K. Bagchi and M. A. Wenger, "Electrophysiological Correlations of Some Yoga Exercises," *Electroencephalography and Clinical Neurophysiology,* 7, 1957, pp. 132–149; and M. A. Wenger, B. K. Bagchi, B. W. Anand, "Experiments in India on 'Voluntary' Control of the Heart and Pulse," *Circulation,* Vol. 24, 1961, pp. 1319–1325.

12. *Be Young with Yoga, op. cit.,* pp. 172–193.

13. B. W. Anand, G. S. Chhina, and B. Singh, "Studies on Shri Ramananda Yogi During His Stay in an Air-Tight Box," *Indian Journal of Medical Research,* 49, 1961, pp. 82–89; and G. V. Satyanarayanamurthi and P. Brahmayyasastry, "A Preliminary Scientific Investigation into Some Unusual Physiological Manifestations Acquired as a Result of Yogic Practices in India," *Vienna Journal of Neurophysiological and Allied Sciences,* 15, 1958, pp. 241–248.

14. K. S. Bhattacharyya and P. Krishnaswami, "Trial of Yogic Exercises," *Armed Forces Medical Journal,* 16, 1960, pp. 222–228; and H. S. Nayar, R. M. Mathur, and R. S. Kumar, "Effects of Yogic Exercise on Human Physical Efficiency," *Indian Journal of Medical Research,* October, 1975, pp. 1369–1376.

15. "Yoga and Fitness," *op. cit.,* p. 27.

16. *Principles of Modern Physical Education, Health, and Recreation, op. cit.,* p. 571.

17. "Experiments in India on 'Voluntary' Control of the Heart and Pulse," *op. cit.,* pp. 1319–1325.

18. "Yoga and Fitness," *op. cit.,* p. 27.

19. *Ibid.*

20. "Effects of Yogic Exercise on Human Physical Efficiency," *op. cit.,* p. 1372.

21. *Ibid.*

22. H. Benson, *The Relaxation Response.* NY: Avon, 1976, pp. 98–99.

23. C. H. Patel, "Yoga and Biofeedback in the Management of Hypertension," *The Lancet,* November 10, 1973.

24. K. K. Datey, S. N. Deshmukh, C. P. Dalvi, and S. L. Vinekar,

"Shavasan: A Yogic Exercise in the Management of Hypertension," *Angiology,* 20, 1969, pp. 325–333.

25. W. Lyon, "Notes on Teaching Yoga," *The Journal of Physical Education,* March/April, 1971, p. 96; and *Executive Fitness Newsletter,* June 16, 1973, p. 3.
26. K. Zebroff and P. Zebroff, *Yoga with Your Children.* Vancouver, British Columbia: Fforbez Enterprises, 1973.
27. *Introduction to Yoga, op. cit.,* pp. 54–100; and *Be Young With Yoga, op. cit.,* p. 155.
28. "Yoga and Fitness," *op. cit.,* p. 26.
29. *Be Young with Yoga, op. cit.* p. 197.
30. *Activetics, op. cit.,* p. 238.
31. R. Hittleman, *Weight Control Through Yoga.* NY: Bantam Books, 1971.

Chapter 13

1. "Masculinity," *Psychology Today,* January, 1977, p. 37.
2. J. H. Wilmore, "Weight Training for Women," *Fitness for Living,* November/December, 1973, p. 44.
3. *Ibid.,* p. 43.
4. M. Yessis, "Relationship Between Varying Combinations of Resistance and Repetitions in the Strength-Endurance Continuum," (unpublished Ph.D. dissertation). Los Angeles, CA: University of Southern California; and "Research and Strength and Development," in J. P. O'Shea (ed.), *Scientific Principles and Methods of Strength Fitness.* Reading, MA: Addison-Wesley, 1976, Chapter 2.
5. C. Atlas, *Dynamic Tension.* NY: Charles Atlas, 1926.
6. T. Hettinger and E. A. Muller, "Muskelleistung und Muskeltraining," *International Zeitschrift für Angewandte Physiologie,* 15, 1953, pp. 111–125.
7. J. G. Crakes, "An Analysis of Some Aspects of an Exercise and Training Program Developed by Hettinger and Muller," (unpublished Master's thesis). Eugene, Oregon: University of Oregon, 1957.
8. D. J. Salls, *Ten Static Exercises.* Annison, AL: Dr. Donald J. Salls Foundation, Inc., 1962.

9. D. W. Mullison, *Isometric Exercises*. Laramie, Wyoming: Ideas Inc., 1964.

10. V. Obeck, *How to Exercise Without Moving a Muscle*. NY: Essandess, 1966.

11. C. Patterson, *Facial Isometrics*. NY: Whiteside, 1964.

12. J. A. Bender, H. M. Kaplan, and A. J. Johnson, "Isometrics: A Critique of Faddism Versus Fact," *Journal of Health, Physical Education, and Recreation*, May, 1963, p. 22.

13. H. Higdon, "Let's Tell The Truth About Isometrics," *Today's Health*, June, 1965, p. 67.

14. "Isometric Exercises May Be Dangerous for Heart Disease Patients," *Journal of American Medical Association*, February 22, 1971, p. 1236.

15. "Isometrics: A Critique of Faddism Versus Fact," *op. cit.*, p. 66.

16. *Individualized Fitness Programs, op. cit.*, p. 123.

17. "Let's Tell the Truth About Isometrics," *op. cit.* p. 66.

18. "Muskelleistung und Muskeltraining," *loc. cit.*

19. "Let's Tell the Truth About Isometrics," *op. cit.*, p. 68.

20. P. H. McHargue, "Reconditioning," p. 406; and H. H. Merrifield, "Rehabilitation," in *The Physical Fitness Encyclopedia, op. cit.*, p. 409.

21. "Isometrics," in *The Physical Fitness Encyclopedia, op. cit.*, pp. 247–248.

22. R. H. Kerber, R. A. Miller, and S. M. Najjar, "Myocardial Ischemic Effects of Isometric, Dynamic and Combined Exercise in Coronary Artery Disease," *Chest*, April, 1975, p. 393.

23. T. L. DeLorme, "Restoration of Muscle Power by Heavy Resistance Exercises," *Journal of Bone, Joint and Surgery*, 37A, 1945, pp. 645–667.

24. R. A. Berger, "Effects of Varied Weight Training Programs on Strength," *Research Quarterly*, 33, 1962, pp. 168–181.

25. H. B. Falls, E. L. Wallis, G. A. Logan, *Foundations of Conditioning*. NY: Academic Press, 1970, p. 72.

26. G. R. Fulton, "Weight Training and Weight Lifting," in *The Physical Fitness Encyclopedia, op. cit.*, p. 541.

27. B. Hoffman, *York Barbell and Dumbbell System* (Courses 1, 2, 3, & 4). York, PA: York Barbell Co., 1946.

28. J. Weider, *Weider's "Triple Progressive" Muscle-Building Courses*. Woodland Hills, CA: Joe Weider, 1975.

29. B. Reynolds, *Complete Weight Training Book*. Mountain View, CA: World Publications, 1976.

30. *The President's Council on Physical Fitness and Sports, Weight Training Program for Strength and Power*. Washington, DC: President's Council on Physical Fitness and Sports (no date).

31. R. B. Parker and J. R. Marsh, *Sports Illustrated's Training with Weights*. Philadelphia, PA: J. B. Lippincott, 1974.

32. L. Ravelle, *Bodybuilding for Everyone*. Buchanan, NY: Emerson Books, Inc., 1975.

33. E. Taylor, *Strength & Stamina Training*. London: John Murray Ltd., 1970.

34. "Weight Training and Weight Lifting," *op. cit.*, p. 539.

35. D. R. Cassidy, D. F. Mapes, L. Alley, *Handbook of Physical Fitness Activities*. NY: Macmillan Co., 1965, p. 52.

36. *The Y's Way to Physical Fitness, op. cit.*, p. 13.

37. "Risks in Weight Lifting" (Letter to the editor), *Journal of American Medical Association*, June 29, 1970, p. 2266.

38. F. E. Jackson, H. J. Sazima, R. A. Pratt, and J. B. Back, "Weight Lifting Injuries," *Journal of American College Health Association*, February, 1971, pp. 187–188.

39. K. K. Klein and W. L. Hall, "The Knee in Athletics," Washington, DC: *American Association for Health and Physical Education*, 1963, pp. 16–20.

40. B. H. Massey, H. W. Freeman, F. R. Manson, and J. A. Wessel, *The Kinesiology of Weight Lifting*. Dubuque, IA: William C. Brown, 1959, p. 8.

41. P. V. Karpovich, "Incidence of Injuries in Weight Lifting," Journal of Physical Education, March/April, 1951, pp. 71–72.

42. *The Kinesiology of Weight Lifting, op. cit.*, p. 4.

43. *Ibid.*, p. 5.

44. *Ibid.*, p. 9.

45. J. J. Perine, "Isokinetic Exercises," *Journal of Health, Physical Education and Recreation*, May, 1968, p. 43.

46. R. Rodale, "A New Exercise Idea," *Fitness For Living*, November/December, 1968, p. 20.

47. H. G. Thistle, *et al.*, "Isokinetic Contractions: A New Concept

of Resistance Exercise," *Archives of Physical Medicine and Rehabilitation*, June, 1967, p. 74.

48. T. V. Pipes and J. H. Wilmore, "Isokınetic Versus Isotonic Strength Training in Adult Men," *Medicine and Science in Sports*, Winter, 1975, p. 262.

49. H. D. Olree, "An Evaluation of the Exer-Genie Exerciser and the Collins Pedal Mode Ergometer for Developing Physical Fitness," NASA Study. NAS-9-9433, 1973, p. 1.

50. *Individualized Fitness Programs, op. cit.,* p. 173.

51. *Ibid.*

52. *Ibid,* p. 125.

Chapter 14

1. R. R. Spackman, Jr., *Exercise in the Office.* Carbondale and Edwardsville, IL: Southern Illinois University Press. 1968, p. v.

2. *Ibid.*

3. O. Graham and C. W. Selin, *Physical Fitness for the Business Man.* Waterford, CT: National Foreman's Institution, 1963.

4. "The New Rx for Better Health," *Business Week,* January 5, 1974, p. 69.

5. *Ibid.*

6. *Weight Control Through Yoga, op. cit.,* p. 7.

7. *Ibid.,* p. 12.

8. *Activetics, op. cit.,* p. 238.

9. J. Mayer, "Should You Starve Yourself Thin?" *Family Health,* February, 1977, p. 24.

10. F. Konishi, *Exercise Equivalents of Food: A Practical Guide for the Overweight.* Carbondale: Southern Illinois University Press, 1974.

11. G. Gwinup, *Energetics: The Key to Weight Control.* Los Angeles, CA: Sherbourne Press, 1970.

12. *Ibid.,* p. 111.

13. F. King and W. F. Herzig, *Golden Age Exercises.* NY: Crown Publishers, 1968.

14. H. A. deVries, *Vigor Regained.* Englewood Cliffs, NJ: Prentice-Hall, 1974.

15. *Ibid.,* p. 84.
16. *The Fitness Challenge . . . in the Later Years.* Washington, DC: President's Council on Physical Fitness and Sports (no date).

Chapter 15

1. "National Adult Physical Fitness Survey," *loc. cit.*
2. C. C. Conrad, "How Different Sports Rate In Promoting Physical Fitness," *Medicine Times,* May, 1976, reprint, pp. 4–5.
3. *Activetics, op. cit.,* p. 225.
4. *Complete Conditioning: The No-Nonsense Guide To Fitness and Good Health, op. cit.,* pp. 145–146.
5. "How Different Sports Rate in Promoting Physical Fitness," *op. cit.,* p. 4.
6. P. D. White, "Forward," in *Cycling.* Washington, DC: American Association of Health, Physical Education and Recreation, 1963.
7. "How Good Is Bike Riding As Primary Exercise?" *The Physician and Sportsmedicine,* May, 1975, p. 41.
8. "How Different Sports Rate in Promoting Physical Fitness," *op. cit.,* p. 2.
9. "How Good Is Bike Riding As Primary Exercise?" *op. cit.,* p. 38.
10. "How Different Sports Rate in Promoting Physical Fitness," *op. cit.,* p. 2.
11. *Activetics, op. cit.,* p. 225.
12. "How Different Sports Rate in Promoting Physical Fitness," *op. cit.,* p. 4.
13. *Activetics, op. cit.,* p. 225.
14. *Complete Conditioning: The No-Nonsense Guide to Fitness and Good Health, op. cit.,* p. 146.
15. "How Different Sports Rate in Promoting Physical Fitness," *op. cit.,* p. 6.
16. *Activetics, op. cit.,* pp. 229–230.
17. *Complete Conditioning: The No-Nonsense Guide to Fitness and Good Health, op. cit.,* p. 145.
18. *Activetics, op. cit.,* p. 230.

19. "How Different Sports Rate in Promoting Physical Fitness," *op. cit.*, p. 3.
20. *Ibid.*, p. 2.
21. *Ibid.*
22. *Ibid.*
23. *Aerobics, op. cit.*
24. *Activetics, op. cit.*, p. 233.
25. "How Different Sports Rate in Promoting Physical Fitness," *op. cit.*, p. 2.
26. "Ice Skating," in *Physical Fitness Encyclopedia, op. cit.*, p. 231.
27. *Activetics, op. cit.*, p. 235.
28. "How Different Sports Rate in Promoting Physical Fitness," *op. cit.*, p. 3.
29. *Ibid.*, p. 4.
30. *Ibid.;* and *Complete Conditioning: The No-Nonsense Guide to Fitness and Good Health, op. cit.*, p. 146.
31. "How Different Sports Rate in Promoting Physical Fitness," *op. cit.*, p. 4.
32. *Activetics, op. cit.*, p. 235.
33. H. A. Hecht, "Skiing," in *Physical Fitness Encyclopedia, op. cit.*, p. 443.
34. *Complete Conditioning: The No-Nonsense Guide to Fitness and Good Health, op. cit.*, p. 146.
35. *Activetics, op. cit.*, p. 235.
36. *Ibid.*, p. 224.
37. "How Different Sports Rate in Promoting Physical Fitness," *op. cit.*, pp. 6–7.
38. T. Irwin, "What Sport Is Best for You," *Family Health*, January, 1975, p. 24.
39. "How Different Sports Rate in Promoting Physical Fitness," *op. cit.*, p. 2.
40. *Ibid.*
41. *Ibid.*, p. 5.
42. *Complete Conditioning: The No-Nonsense Guide to Physical Fitness and Good Health, op. cit.*, pp. 144–145.
43. "How Different Sports Rate in Promoting Physical Fitness," *op. cit.*, p. 5.
44. *Ibid.*, p. 7.

45. M. L. Walters, "Volleyball," in *Physical Fitness Encyclopedia, op. cit.,* pp. 518–519.
46. C. R. Meyers, "Water Skiing," in *Physical Fitness Encyclopedia, op. cit.,* pp. 528–529.
47. *Ibid.,* p. 529.
48. "How Different Sports Rate in Promoting Physical Fitness," *op. cit.,* p. 7.

Chapter 16

1. "Exercise Equipment—The Good, the Bad and the Ugly," *Fitness For Living,* March/April, 1971, p. 25.
2. R. Sherrill, "Before You Believe Those Exercise and Diet Ads, Read the Following Report," *Today's Health,* August, 1971, p. 34; and "Exercise Equipment—The Good, the Bad and the Ugly," *op. cit.*
3. "Exercise Equipment—The Good, the Bad and the Ugly," *op. cit.,* p. 26.
4. Editors of *Consumer Reports, The Medicine Show.* Mount Vernon, NY: Consumers Union, 1970, p. 115.
5. A. Steinhaus and V. Heinlund, "Do Mechanical Vibrators Take Off or Redistribute Fat?" *Journal of Association for Physical and Mental Rehabilitation,* 11:1957, p. 3.
6. *The Medicine Show, op. cit.,* pp. 115–116.

Chapter 17

1. "Man, Sweat, and Performance" (pamphlet), Rutherford, NJ: Becton, Dickinson and Co., 1969; and C. T. Kuntzleman, "Sweat to Save Your Life," *Fitness for Living,* September/ October, 1970, pp. 24–25.
2. "Man, Sweat, and Performance," *op. cit.;* and *Keep Your Heart Running, op. cit.,* p. 194.
3. *The Official YMCA Physical Fitness Handbook, op. cit.,* p. 78.
4. *Total Fitness, op. cit.,* p. 43.
5. *Ibid.,* p. 43.

6. *Ibid.*, p. 44.
7. *The Y's Way to Physical Fitness, op. cit.*, p. 18.
8. J. Hansen, M. Karvonen, and P. Piironen, "Physiological Effects of Extreme Heat as Studied in the Finnish Sauna Bath," *American Journal of Physical Medicine*, 45:1966 and 46:1967.
9. H. deVries, P. Beckmann, H. Hubert, and L. Dieckmeir, "Electromyographic Evaluation of the Effects of Sauna on the Neuromuscular System," *Journal of Sports Medicine and Physical Education*, 8:1961, p. 61.
10. M. L. Lehtments, "The Sauna Bath, History, Development and Physiological Effects," *International Review of Physical Medicine and Rehabilitation*, 36:1957, pp. 21-64.
11. "Sweating It Out Helps Clear Uremia," *Medical World News*, April 29, 1966, p. 12.
12. "The Sauna Bath, History, Development and Physiological Effects," *op. cit.*
13. R. C. Warner, "Sauna Baths: A Review of the Literature" (pamphlet). NY: Greater YMCA of New York, 1971, p. 16.
14. M. Karvonen, O. Friberg, and E. Antilla, "Urine Flow and Water Balance in the Sauna Bath," *Annals of Medicine and Experimental Biology*, 35:1955, p. 326.
15. H. Johnson, "Staying Healthy—Will Sauna Baths Improve Your Health?" (pamphlet). NY: Life Extension Institute, 1964.
16. "Sauna Baths: A Review of the Literature," *op. cit.*, p. 15.
17. B. Saltin, "Circulatory Response to Submaximal and Maximal Exercise After Thermal Dehydration," *Journal of Applied Physiology*, 9:1964, p. 1125.
18. "Physiological Effects of Extreme Heat As Studied in the Finnish Sauna Bath," *loc. cit.*,
19. "Sauna Baths: A Review of the Literature," *op. cit.*, p. 15.
20. "Sauna Baths May Imperil Elderly or Sick Bathers," *Medical Tribune*, October 12, 1970, p. 11.
21. *Activetics, op. cit.*, p. 38.
22. *Ibid.*, p. 40.
23. C. MacIntyre, "These Inflatable Outfits—Do They Really Work?" *Fitness For Living*, March/April, 1973, pp. 38-40.

24. *The Y's Way to Physical Fitness, op. cit.,* p. 18.
25. "Editor's Note," *Fitness For Living,* March/April, 1973, p. 41.

Chapter 18

1. "The Influence of Exercise on the Morphology and Metabolism of the Isolated Fat Cell," symposium presented at the 20th Annual Meeting of the American College of Sports Medicine, May 7, 1973, Seattle, Washington. Chairman Charles M. Tipton.
2. V. P. Dole, "Energy Storage," in A. E. Renold and G. F. Cahill, Jr. (eds.), *Adipose Tissue.* Washington, DC: American Physiological Society, 1965, p. 13.
3. J. Vague and R. Fenasse, "Comparative Anatomy of Adipose Tissue," in *Adipose Tissue,* pp. 35–36.
4. *Ibid.*
5. *Overweight: Causes, Cost, and Control, op. cit.,* pp. 66–67.
6. J. L. Knittle, "Obesity in Childhood: A Problem in Adipose Tissue Cellular Development," *Journal of Pediatrics,* 81:1972, p. 1053.
7. "Comparative Anatomy of Adipose Tissue," in *Adipose Tissue, op. cit.,* pp. 35–36.
8. "Obesity in Childhood: A Problem in Adipose Tissue Cellular Development," *op. cit.,* p. 1054.
9. "Is Massage Good For You?" *Fitness For Living,* November/December, 1968, p. 62.
10. M. E. Knapp, "Massage," *Postgraduate Medicine,* July, 1968, p. 193.
11. *Ibid.*
12. B. Prudden, *How to Keep Slender and Fit After 30.* NY: Pocket Books, 1970, p. 51.
13. A. H. Steinhaus and V. Henlund, "Do Mechanical Vibrators Take Off Or Redistribute Fat?" *Journal of Association for Physical and Mental Rehabilitation,* 11:1957, p. 3.
14. N. Ronsard, *Cellulite: Those Lumps, Bumps, and Bulges You Couldn't Lose Before.* NY: Beauty and Health Pub. Co., 1973.
15. N. Ronsard, *Cellulite.* NY: Bantam, 1975, p. 19.

16. *Ibid.*, p. 22.

17. *Ibid.*

18. A. Eugene, *Say Goodbye to Cellulite* (Opa Locka, FL: Improvement Books, 1974); Carol Ann Rinsler, *Banish Those Unsightly Cellulite Bumps Forever!* (NY: Pocket Books, 1975); and Susan Winer, *How to Be Cellulite Free Forever.* NY: Dell, 1975).

19. *Activetics, op. cit.,* p. 42.

20. *Ibid.*

21. *Complete Conditioning, op. cit.,* p. 122.

22. H. E. Wertheimer, "Introduction—A Perspective," in *Adipose Tissue, op. cit.,* pp. 5–6.

23. R. Lindsey, "Figure Wrapping: Can You Believe It?" *Fitness For Living,* March/April, 1972, p. 57.

24. *Ibid.*

25. *Ibid.*

26. *Ibid.*, p. 59.

27. *Ibid.*

Chapter 19

1. "How America Gets into Shape," *Datsun Action,* Issue 1, 1976, p. 10.

2. J. N. Tuck, "Health Clubs: Fit to Be Tried by Your Patients?" *The Physician and Sportsmedicine,* September, 1976, p. 112.

3. D. Moore, "When Better Bodies Are Built . . . ," *Consumer Survival Kit,* Maryland Center for Public Broadcasting, 1976, p. 10.

4. "Health Clubs: Fit to Be Tried by Your Patients?" *op. cit.,* p. 114.

5. "Deception Is Laid to 11 Health Spas," *The New York Times,* Wednesday, July 17, 1974, p. 73.

6. "The FTC Proposes Curbs on Health Clubs," *Washington Post,* August 16, 1973.

7. *Ibid.*

8. "When Better Bodies Are Built . . . ," *op. cit.,* p. 16.

9. Association of Physical Fitness Centers, *The Health Spa Industry: A Private-Sector Solution to a National Problem.* Towson, Maryland (no date), p. 6.

10. "How America Gets Into Shape," *op. cit.,* p. 10.

11. E. Buckley (ed.), *1974 YMCA Yearbook,* Vol. 2. New York: National Council of YMCAs, 1974, pp. 267–268; 302–304; and 378–379.

INDEX

A selection of books published by Penguin is listed on the following pages.

For a complete list of books available from Penguin in the United States, write to Dept. DG, Penguin Books, 299 Murray Hill Parkway, East Rutherford, New Jersey 07073.

For a complete list of books available from Penguin in Canada, write to Penguin Books Canada Limited, 2801 John Street, Markham, Ontario L3R 1B4.

SWIMMING SKILLS
Freestyle, Butterfly, Backstroke, Breaststroke

Dr. Frank Ryan

With swimming more popular now than ever before, Dr. Frank Ryan brings his acclaimed expertise in sports technique to the four competitive strokes: freestyle, backstroke, breaststroke, and the strenuous and spectacular butterfly stroke. The emphasis is on those methods of physical and mental conditioning that not only make world champions but also make the rest of us go through the water a little faster. Dr. Ryan details the mechanics of achieving form, power, speed, and endurance. His book, illustrated with many photographs and diagrams, unites the latest and most innovative theories with the experience and concern of the successful coach.

WEIGHT TRAINING

Dr. Frank Ryan

Weight training, as opposed to weight lifting, is an invaluable aid in preparing for almost every sport. The goal of weight training is to develop coordinated power—the ability of a muscle, group of muscles, or the body itself to go farther or longer, run faster or harder, jump higher or wider. Stressing the need for safety and protection from injuries, acclaimed sports expert Dr. Frank Ryan covers each step in the process of physical development and coordination through exercise with weights and shows how this process can lead to athletic excellence.

THE RUNNER'S HANDBOOK
A Complete Fitness Guide for Men and Women on the Run

Bob Glover and Jack Shepherd

Here is the indispensable guide, with the simple secrets of success, for all runners and would-be runners. Bob Glover's Run-Easy Method adapts to beginners of all ages but will also benefit those at intermediate and more advanced levels. A veteran marathoner, Glover includes advice on competing in races up to and beyond the full 26.2-mile marathon distance, and he clarifies the sometimes confusing training methods and diets. He and Jack Shepherd discuss the fine points of running style, stretching exercises and weight training, selecting shoes and other equipment, preparing for weather and road conditions, and avoiding injury when you can and coping with it when you can't (Glover claims firsthand knowledge of almost every injury that can strike a runner!). They take a quick look at the new field of running and meditation and a longer look at the effects of running on the heart and lungs—information and advice garnered from many of the country's top running doctors. A guide to running spaces in more than twenty-five major American cities is also included.

THE RUNNER'S HANDBOOK TRAINING DIARY

Bob Glover and Jack Shepherd

Over thirty million Americans run every day for fitness and health. As these runners improve their speed, increase their mileage, and reach out toward racing, they will want to keep a systematic account of runs, time, weather, running paths, distances, conditioning, and other important facets of their training. Now the authors of *The Runner's Handbook* have provided such a record, including a week-at-a-glance section, fifty-two weeks with space for all relevant data; running tips for each season; charts and training tips for beginning, intermediate, and advanced runners; advice on how to return to running after an injury or illness; and much more. *The Runner's Handbook Training Diary* is today's most indispensable tool for men and women on the run.

THE EYE BOOK

John Eden, M.D.

How much do you really know about your eyes? Can reading in dim light injure your vision? Are cheap sunglasses bad for your eyes? Will eye exercises improve nearsightedness, farsightedness, and other eye problems? Do contact lenses prevent nearsightedness from progressing? Is sitting too close to a movie or television screen harmful? The answer to all these questions is no. In *The Eye Book* Dr. John Eden demolishes these myths and many other widespread misconceptions, explaining in clear language how eyes work, how to maintain their health, what can go wrong with them, and how to deal with ocular difficulties and diseases—and he also explores the newest innovations in first-aid technique, surgical procedures, and contact lenses.

MEDICAL ADVANCES

Lawrence Galton

Here is a book that brings to the layman some of the latest developments in medical research, including three hundred new treatments for major and minor ailments such as breast cancer, depression, hay fever, headaches, acne, arthritis, diabetes, ulcers, heartburn, insomnia, and hundreds of other afflictions. Lawrence Galton reports on the newest discoveries all over the medical world. Many of these advances are based on breakthroughs so recent that most people—even doctors—have not yet read about them. The treatments are meticulously footnoted to enable your doctor to refer to technical sources so that the scientific evidence can be weighed. *Medical Advances* is intended to encourage patients to work with their physicians in finding and applying the most useful techniques of today's medicine.